INTERMITTENT

FASTING

Complete Step-By-Step Guide to lose weight quickly, slow aging and increase quality of life through the process of metabolic autophagy.

Includes: Meal Plans with more than 80 Delicious Recipes.

BY MELANY FLORES

CONTENTS

INTRODUCTION

I want to thank you and congratulate you on choosing this book.

Undoubtedly, intermittent fasting is making headlines for all the right reasons. It has become popular over the years, because of its ability to assist women on their weight loss journey. This particular diet regime does not only help women to lose weight, but it can also bless them with a range of other benefits. It can boost their heart's health, keeps them away from cancer and diabetes, and also takes care of their brain.

One of the many reasons why intermittent fasting has become so popular is because it is so much easier to follow than other diets. It doesn't keep you deprived of eating. All you need to do is follow a set schedule of eating, and you are good to go.

In this book, I will guide you through various methods of intermittent fasting. I will explain to you how this entire concept works. Additionally, I will provide you with some delicious meal plans.

So, let's get started!

Don't forget to leave a short review of this book on Amazon if you enjoy it, I'd love to hear your opinion!

WHAT IS INTERMITTENT FASTING?

Weight loss and intermittent fasting (IF) actually go hand in hand. Do not believe us? Read this: a recent report revealed that intermittent fasting is very effective for weight loss and can cause a loss of nearly 7-11 pounds over a period of 10 weeks.

Doesn't that sound great?

Undoubtedly, IF is the best way to lose weight. Intermittent fasting is healthier and relatively easierthan the usual methods of fasting.

Here is an obvious question – what is intermittent fasting, anyway?

Intermittent fasting essentially comprises a pattern of eating that alternates between fasting and eating. Unlike a typical diet, intermittent fasting does not dictate what kinds of food one should eat. Instead, it focuses on the timing of the consumption of food.

The entire process focuses more on WHEN you eat the food rather thanWHAT you eat. Therefore, this is not a very typical dieting regime. In fact, it works more as an eating pattern.

There are many ways to carry out intermittent fasting. For instance you could adopt a daily 16-hour fasting streak or a 24-hour fasting streak carried out mainly for two days a week.

What are the different types of intermittent fasting?

16/8 method

This is the most popular IF method for losing weight. It is also known as the Leangains protocol.

It involves a 16-hour fasting period. This means that all your meals must take place in the remaining eight hours of the day. If you start your meals at 1 pm, you should be able to complete all your meals by 9pm. According to the 16/8 method, you must also skip breakfast on a regular basis. Thus, whatever you eat during the course of the day should be restricted to that 8-hour timeline.

Eat-stop-eat method

This method differs slightly from the 16/8 method. Instead of fasting for 16 hours, you should fast for about 24 hours. For instance, if you start the fasting process by skipping dinner for one day, then you should continue to fast until the dinner meal the next day. However, this fasting process should be done only once or twice a week. The eat-stop-eat fasting method is easier than the 16/8 method because it is less frequent.

5:2 diet

The last type of intermittent fasting, the 5:2 diet, includes fasting for about two days a week and eating normally during other days of the week.

However, this type of fasting involves certain complications. For instance, you must only consume a maximum of 500 to 600 calories per day.

This method should be adopted twice a week but on two non-consecutive days. For instance, if you fast on Monday, you would have to eat normally on Tuesday and then you could fast on any other day of the week.

Essentially, each of these three methods contributes heavily to individual weight loss and can help you to maintain body fitness. This is because all the IF methods focus on restricting the amount of calorie intake.

However, the most popular method for intermittent fasting is the 16/8 method. It is the most convenient method since the fasting and eating periods remain the same length of time on each day of the week.

WHAT EFFECT DOES INTERMITTENT FASTING HAVE ON YOUR BODY'S CELLS AND HORMONES ?

There is a reason why intermittent fasting is the favorite method of weight loss, particularly for women. It does not dictate what you should eat. It tells you when to eat and when not to eat. Essentially, you alternate between eating and fasting until you achieve your desired weight.

But have you wondered how this unique approach works? Your body goes through thousands of changes when you adopt an IF method. All the cells and hormones inside you start working differently when they receive food in a dissimilar fashion than before. Your body ensures that the stored fat is more accessible during your fasting periods.

Keep reading to learn how your body loses weight with IF.

Reduction insulin levels

It is worth mentioning here that high levels of insulin can be dangerous for your body. These high insulin levels could trigger several types of illnesses. However, fasting can improve the body's insulin sensitivity and reduce the body's levels of insulin. Once these insulin levels are reduced, the fat stored in the body becomes more accessible; therefore, it can be burned more easily. This results in weight loss, which is one of the primary benefits offered by intermittent fasting.

Enhanced genes

The body's genes are also positively impacted by the process of intermittent fasting. When the body does not have access to new fat regularly, the genes tend to work on themselves. The functional role of the genes undergoes some modification due to which their longevity increases and they become more capable of a solid defense mechanism. This means that they can protect the body against the outside germs and diseases which, in turn, boosts the immunity level of the body.

Reduction in insulin resistance

Most diets do not focus on developing the body's insulin resistance. However, this is essential because even if you start losing weight, high insulin resistance will keep your insulin levels high. You might not be able to go too far only by burning fat to get energy. Fasting is a great way to decrease this resistance.

Now you know that the level of the hormone insulin undergoes changes. In addition to burning the fat, this reduced insulin resistance lowers the risk of type-2 diabetes and increases your metabolism. IF is used as a top remedy for those facing high blood sugar problems.

Cut down on oxidative stress

Oxidative stress is when harmful free radicals move around your body to damage important molecules. It is increased when there is a lack of antioxidants in the body to detoxify its effects. This stress contributes to aging and many chronic diseases.

These unstable molecules damage the proteins and DNA in your body. But research has shown that intermittent fasting increases the body's resistance to oxidative stress. Thus, you get to lose weight and save yourself from serious diseases too.

Better heart health

High insulin levels lead to high blood pressure, high cholesterol levels, and obesity, which all increase your chances of developing heart disease. Cholesterol levels are also directly linked to inflammation caused by metabolic syndrome (the plaque build-up in the arteries).

When your insulin levels drop during fasting periods, all the above numbers come down. And you, therefore, reduce the risk for cardiovascular (in short, heart) diseases. A healthy heart is always preferable.

Faster cell repair process

Fasting triggers autophagy, which is a waste removal process initiated by the cells in your body. When you fast, the broken and dysfunctional proteins that build up in the cells start metabolizing. The cells break down and remove all unwanted materials inside them. This helps them undergo a much quicker repair process.

May prevent cancer and Alzheimer's disease

The above process that cells undergo while fasting does more than repair cells more quickly. The removal of harmful waste from the cells protects against harmful diseases like cancer and Alzheimer's. In women, intermittent fasting has been known to reduce the risk of breast cancer.

Increased brain function

The reduction in oxidative stress, inflammation, and blood sugar levels are all important for your brain health. Also, IF is known to increase the production of new brain cells, or the neurons which benefit the brain function.

Brain-derived neurotrophic factor (BDNF) is a hormone in the brain whose deficiency is known to be associated with depression and other brain problems. Intermittent fasting increases the levels of BDNF.

Off-balance menstrual cycle

Women need certain nutrients and calories to stay on track with their menses. Their hypothalamic–pituitary–gonadal axis does not get enough support when there is a substantial decrease in calories. The initial months of intermittent fasting could throw off the menstrual cycle in some women. Thus, it is highly recommended to consult your doctor before proceeding with this regime.

More leptin, less ghrelin

Ghrelin is a hormone that tells you when you are hungry. Leptin is the "I am full" hormone of your body that makes you sense satiety. Both of them are directly related to your food intake.

Intermittent fasting increases the leptin levels and lowers the ghrelin levels in the body. As a result, you feel fuller faster and hungry less often. This simply translates to consuming fewer calories and as a result, weight loss.

Pregnancy support

Fasting greatly affects a woman's reproductive cycle. If your body does not receive enough nutritional and metabolic energy to carry out a pregnancy, your body signals the brain to shut down the reproductive cycle.

Therefore, it becomes essential to be careful about fasting if you are trying to get pregnant. Your diet should have a high nutritional profile, and the calorie restrictions should not be strict. You would need the full support of your body to get pregnant.

As a combination of all these factors, that includes the burning of stored fat, the repair of cells, and the functions of the genes, intermittent fasting proves to be a very effective solution in maintaining the overall health of the body. However, the primary reason why people approach this type of eating habit is basically because of its massive weight loss capabilities.

BENEFITS OF INTERMITTENT FASTING

Intermittent fasting is making headlines, because of the range of benefits that it provides. In this section, we will examine these benefits in greater detail.

Intermittent Fasting leads to Weight Loss

For any diet or weight loss method to work, you must monitor your calorie intake either you must consume fewer calories daily or burn them off regularly. Thus, all the fasting methods focus on reducing the number of calories that you consume.

If you skip certain meals intermittently, you consume fewer calories. For example, if you skip breakfast in the morning, you decrease your daily calorie intake by 500 calories. That is how intermittent fasting causes weight loss.

1. Intermittent fasting leads to the loss of body fat.

You might say that you want to lose weight. However, it is not the weight that you should focus on, but the extra body fat. This is important to mention because weight loss could also be triggered by a loss of muscle mass. However, that is not something you would want to achieve.

The idea is to get rid of excess body fat and not muscle mass. Losing muscle mass actually does not serve the purpose here. According to various studies, intermittent fasting helps you lose excess body fat rather than muscle mass. This is how it contributes to effective weight loss.

2.   Intermittent fasting preserves muscle mass

Most of the weight loss routines available to us focus on losing both muscle mass and excess body fat. Losing muscle mass is undesirable because it could lead to dropping metabolic rates that could be harmful to your body.

3.   Intermittent fasting can keep you from gaining weight during the holidays.

Weight gain is a steady process that occurs throughout the year. However, around the time of holidays like Christmas and Thanksgiving, and other vacation periods, the rate of weight gain increases dramatically!

This is the time when intermittent fasting could really help you. In fact, in these situations, alternate periods of eating and fasting could keep your calorie count in check and you do not have to worry about eating big for the other meals. So, even during your holidays, you could maintain a rather simple diet of intermittent fasting and you are good to go!

4.   Intermittent fasting does not result in

extreme hunger cravings

Unlike other fasting methods and techniques, intermittent fasting does notcause severe hunger cravings, which might cause you to overeat. Intermittent fasting controls your diet and hunger, so,you would be able to eat less without having major hunger cravings.

How does intermittent fasting control your hanger? IF keeps your hunger hormones at bay. Thus, they do not affect your body adversely.

What Do Studies Say?

An average human being must lose about 1600-1800 calories per day to lose weight. By skipping breakfast as a part of intermittent fasting, 30% of that target is already achieved.

Studies suggest that IF causes weight loss of about 4-7% near the waist circumference across a period of 24 weeks. This results in the loss of belly fat.

Usually, other dieting methods and restrictions can get rid of 25% of muscle mass but this is harmful to the body and not recommended. In contrast, intermittent fasting can remove only about 10% of muscle mass.

According to studies, fasting regularly causeshunger hormones to run into overdrive. However, since intermittent fasting requires you to alternate periods of fasting and eating, you do not get hunger cravings.

INTERMITTENT FASTING REDUCES THE RISK OF TYPE 2 DIABETES

Each person is unique with a unique combination and type of body structure. Thus, different people react differently to diabetes issues and symptoms. In effect, there are several different ways of treating type2 diabetes.

However, intermittent fasting is known to be more effective than other methods when it comes to reducing the risks of type 2 diabetes. Alternate periods of fasting and eating, help reduce the imbalance of glucose in the body.

What Do Studies Suggest?

It has been noted that people who restrict their diets by consuming their food only during certain times of the day while fasting during the rest of the day (while fasting during the rest of the day), seem to maintain their glucose levels more successfully.

If you consume your calories for the day during only certain times of the day for a period of eight days your insulin sensitivity will increase significantly. This will be accompanied by an increased pancreatic response to changing insulin levels. The earlier that you finish your meals, the greater the likelihood that your body will be at reduced risk of developing several different diseases. Furthermore, you will benefit from a reduction in blood pressure, oxidative stress and even reduced hunger cravings.

It is not enough to consume all your meals as early as possible. It is important to ensure that to meal timings are synchronized with the body's natural biological clock

There aremany underlying benefits and concepts associated with intermittent fasting and its impact on type 2 diabetes. Controlling the glucose levels within the body is more convenient in the morning than in the evening. Thus, intermittent fasting, carried out during the morning (across eight hours) allows you to control the sugar content in the body more easily.

Many studies have been conducted in the recent past that explain the effect of intermittent fasting on maintaining the glucose levels in the body. On such study included research on eight men with prediabetes.

In this particular study, the eight men were asked to eat their breakfast between 6:30 and 8:30 a.m. Thereafter, they were provided with a 6-hour time frame during which they would have to finish the rest of the meals. They were required to fast during the rest of the day and not were not allowed to eat anything while carrying out their normal activities. As a result, all of them managed to finish their dinner by 3 p.m.

There was a second group involved in the same study. This group maintained their diet across a 12-hour time frame. They managed to eat the same kind of foods, at regular intervals.

The researchers found that the first group of people, the ones who could finish the entire diet within the 6-hour period had better insulin sensitivity.

What's more, it was also found that the pancreas reacts better to rising levels of insulin in the body. As a combination of these two factors, the body becomes better equipped to deal with varying levels of glucose.

The benefits of intermittent fasting do not end there. It has been observed that this type of diet reduces blood pressure in men.

Intermittent fasting decreases the risk of developing type 2 diabetes and hypertension. These health benefits, coupled with weight loss, illustrate how intermittent fasting is great for your overall health.

Intermittent Fasting Enhances Brain Health

Let us begin this discussion by finding out what studies have discovered.

A study was conducted on mice where one was given free access to food while the other was kept on a brief intermittent fasting diet. It was found that the latter learned better and retained a better memory than the former one.

Another study using animals showed that intermittent fasting helps reduce inflammation in the brain and helps to lower the risk of many neurological disorders, (including Alzheimer's, and Parkinson's) and the risk of strokes.

These studies used animals and mammals, but some of the results can be applied to human beings. Neuroscience research has supported the fact that IF helps your brain in many ways. Some of them have been listed below.

Making BDNF

Brain-derived neurotrophic factor(BDNF) is an essential protein present in the brain that is responsible for the growth of new neurons. It enhances the communication process within the brain, and acts as a natural antidepressant.

Not just that, BDNF also helps the neurons to stay healthy for a longer time. Dementia, Alzheimer's and other brain-related problems are linked directly to low levels of BDNF in the brain.

Intermittent fasting increases the production of these proteins. A 400 increase in BDNF levels has been observed in people following IF.

Anti-Aging Effects

A group of ten people with cognitive impairment (loss of ability to think, recollect and memorize) were chosen for research. They had started showing early signs of Alzheimer's. Some changes were made to their lifestyle, one of which was to fast for 12-14 hours every night. After 3-6 months, nine out of the ten subjects had improved their cognitive abilities.

This study demonstrates that IF keeps your brain younger. It protects against the loss of structure and function of neurons. The slow-down of neurodegeneration also slows down the aging of the brain. You stay smarter and mentally active for a longer time if you fast regularly.

Seizure Reduction

Carbohydrates are considered the main fuel for the brain. Reports suggest that the brain uses more carbs when you are fasting than when you are not fasting. This leads to a significant reduction in the number of epileptic seizures. Therefore, IF plays a crucial role in decreasing the risk for epilepsy and abnormal functioning of the brain.

Decreased Brain Damage

Studies have shown that fasting increases BDNF, anti-oxidant and anti-inflammatory compounds in the brain. It also decreases brain damage and most importantly, protects a person from dying from a stroke. This is a big advantage that comes by simply opting for scheduled eating time. Since intermittent fasting only tells you to eat in a particular window in a day, the benefits that come along are much greater. Anyone would wish to prevent brain damage for as long as possible.

Improved Brain Function

Think about how exercise affects your muscles. Even a little workout makes them more efficient and healthier. The same thing happens with your brain when you are fasting. The brain cells are put under mild stress, which causes them to slowly adapt to the environment they are being forced into. This makes them more energy efficient and active.

Your body recovers from intense exercise by burning the extra fat and cleansing the cells. The brain does recover from fasting by entering the building phase. This improves brain function and neuronal connections.

Higher HGH

Human growth hormone (HGH) provides the following benefits to the human body:

- Powerful anti-aging properties

- Longevity

- Neurogenesis (making new nerve cells and tissues)

- Neuroprotection

- Cognition

- Cell repair

- The health of brain cells

When a hormone is this essential for your body, it is sensible to focus on generating it at high levels. Intermittent fasting naturally boosts the HGH levels in your body. Taking this hormone from outside artificial sources is not the best for your body and is not recommended for a lot of reasons.

More Energy

You would know that mitochondria are known as the powerhouse of the cells. Each cell contains thousands of mitochondria that give them the power to carry out the body's functions. They are work like the batteries in your phone. Higher battery storage makes your phone last longer and works more efficiently. A higher number of mitochondria in the brain cells means more brain-power.

Studies have shown that intermittent fasting boosts mitochondrial biogenesis, the creation of new mitochondria.

Fasting results in several positive neurochemical changes in the brain cells that improve the cognitive function. Restricting calorie intake reduces inflammation in the brain and increases the production and growth of neurons in the brain. This is a big factor behind increasing your learning power and memory capacity. Studies have also indicated that fasting increases the ability of nerve cells to repair DNA.

Intermittent fasting doesn't just lead to weight loss and a healthy heart; it enhances brain health and function.

Intermittent Fasting Takes Care of Your Heart

Based on a report published by the WHO (World Health Organization), each year, 17.9 million people around the world die due to cardiovascular diseases. This is about one-third of all deaths that occur in a year in the world. This shows that heart diseases are a serious problem today. People over the age of 45 years are affected the most by them.

Modifiable factors such as smoking, obesity, lack of physical activity, metabolism disorders, hypertension, poor diet, andhigh cholesterol, are some of the major factors that lead to the development of serious heart diseases in individuals. We call them modifiable because certain changes in a person's lifestyle can reduce the related risk. These changes include making adjustments like smoking cessation, increasing physical activity and maintaining proper body weight.

Obese people are usually the target of heart-related problems. Studies have found that fighting obesity can be a solution to all of them and it can be achieved by reducing a person's calorie intake and burning their extra-fat. The easiest way to achieve this is through intermittent fasting methods, which mainly focus on consuming meals within a strictly defined period.

It has been confirmed that an IF diet enhances the health of a person's heart. A healthy heart means longevity and a healthy body. This is due to the impact that IF has on various factors that increase the risk of catching a cardiovascular disease. Some of the major impacts have been discussed below:

Lowers Blood Pressure

High level of blood pressure, also known as hypertension, is the main reason behind a stroke or chronic kidney disease. Research and experiments have shown that fasting can help to reduce blood pressure.

Regular intake of high-calorie food leads to increased weight, cholesterol, and blood pressure. Strict dieting methods help to reduce the number of calories a person consumes daily. Intermittent fasting gives the body a long time to use the extra calories to provide energy to the body.

When you alternate eating with fasting, your body's food cravings decrease. Your body burns its excess calories to boost your metabolism and give you energy.

Lower blood pressure levels prevent any sort of heart problems from developing.

Reduces Cholesterol

The risk of having a heart attack is high in individuals with elevated cholesterol levels. These people who regularly consume oily and fries items, for example.

The human body undergoes a lot of internal transformations while fasting. Its metabolic processes improve. Various studies show that the level of total cholesterol (TC) triglycerides and low-density cholesterol (LDL) decrease when a person is fasting. This, in turn, results in limiting the risk of developing coronary heart disease.

Controls Diabetes

Diabetes is caused when the blood sugar levels and insulin resistance in person's body are dangerously high. Intermittent fasting improves blood sugar control, which is useful for those who are at risk of developing diabetes.

When you follow the 'fast and feast' method, insulin resistance decreases, and it becomes easier for the insulin to transport glucose from the blood to the cells more efficiently. Keeping the blood sugar and insulin levels under control goes a long way in ensuring a healthy heart.

Reduces Inflammation

Low levels of inflammation are very helpful for better health. A study performed on 50 healthy adults showed that one month of intermittent fasting decreased their inflammatory markers by a considerable amount. Although acute inflammation is a normal immune process, too much of anything is always harmful. That is why chronic levels may lead to the development of heart diseases.

Decreases the Risk of Metabolic Syndrome

Metabolic syndrome happens when a combination of conditions (high blood pressure, high blood sugar, high cholesterol, excess body fat) come together as a cluster. This increases the risk of heart disease, stroke or type 2 diabetes.

The whole process of intermittent fasting is effective because it burns the extra fat and mass stored in the body. This, in turn, greatly helps in maintaining a healthy cardiovascular system. All these positive changes change the concentration of metabolic biomarkers in the body, thus reducing the risk of metabolic syndrome.

A Healthy Heart is Important

The mortality rate is different in males and females. Studies show that the death rate is higher in men between the age of 45 and 59, while in women it becomes dominant after the age of 60. This is due to the effect of menopause on woman's heart.

All the causes of an unhealthy heart are linked to each other. Excessive fat, high cholesterol, increased blood pressure and sugar levels trigger one other. If one number changes, it causes others to change as well. Though this is bad for your health, you can turn this dependency upside down to your advantage. When you are fasting, your body looks for energy sources to boost metabolic activities. This is when the stored fat of your body comes into play. It is broken down and the energy in it is used by the blood.

When this fat burns, it decreases all other factors leading to an unhealthy heart. Even during your non-fasting period, you should eat food that regulates digestion and contributes to better heart health.

Choose a nutritional diet that helps to diminish the level of your body fat. Doing this will help you to losing weight and prevent you from becoming obese. In short, intermittent fasting is a good way to ensure that you have a healthy heart.

THE TRUTH ABOUT INTERMITTENT FASTING

With all the rage, support, trendiness, and glamour associated with Intermittent Fasting, it's uncomplicated to get up and seek the truth behind all of it. After all, when you are looking forward to giving up your comfort zone and dedicatedly devote yourself to such a strict eating regime, you need to be sure about the results or pay-outs. You need to be sure that it's worth pursuing and is not just another millennial fad.

So, here are some answers to your intriguing questions:

Is it even safe?

Intermittent fasting isn't a new fad. It has been around for years. In the Hindu religion, certain festivals require devotees to refrain from eating for the entireday. Ramadan is an Islamic holy month during which people don't consume food from sunrise to sunset. In Christianity, fasting occurs during Lent. So, it's safe to say that people have been practicing intermittent fasting in the past, and it hasn't caused any major serious complications.

Your body has enough energy stored in the fat cells to get you through the day without food and water. This won't even cause any major hormone imbalances either, thanks to the magical adaptability of our body when under stress.

But to ensure complete safety, you should pick the IF type that's suited to your body. If you're overweight, an 8-hour fast is always better than a 24-hour fast or 5:2 IF. Additionally, it's important to refuel your body with essential proteins, vitamins, minerals and lots of water after you finish fasting. This will ensure your body returns to normal and starts functioning the way it's supposed to.

Will I get too weak?

The simple answer is no. As stated previously, your body has stored enough calories in the fatty cells to get you through the fasting hours. When you fast, your body enters a state known as gluconeogenesis. This is when the liver creates its own glucose to keep your body running. You maytemporarily experience dizziness, or fatigue (which is completely normal). Many professional athletes and experienced dieters even perform physical activities and hit the gym while fasting. So, you shouldn't be worrying about weakness.

How does it affect my metabolism?

Many people believe that IF negatively affectstheir metabolism. But when you lose weight, the body adapts and causes your metabolism to slow down. This is because losing weight is accompanied by the loss of muscle and fat, which provide the required calories during the fasting hours.

Your body goes into fasting mode only after 8 hours of fasting, when it enters the gluconeogenesis state. At this point, there is no glucose left in the liver, and the fat reserves are used. It is only after 24 to 48 hours that your body goes into starvation mode and over time, the metabolic rate decreases. The body does this as a defense mechanism.

Some studies have indicated that in the long-term, calorie restriction reduces the metabolic rate, but any major or minor complications are almost non-existent. More quality research is required to determinate the long-term effects of IF on metabolic rate, but until now it's been on the safe side.

Will it help me to lose weight?

All the protocols of IF should be diligently followed and correctly timed in order to ensure weight loss.

For example, when using the 16:8 intermittent fasting method, you should only consume food during the 8 hour window and fast for the remaining 16 hours. As a rule, you also need to refrain from eating, processed junk food, which can increase your calories.

While it definitely is a safe option for weight loss when done correctly, its effectiveness is still under scrutiny. Some studies have pointed out that it is an excellent weight-loss method, while others have found no significant cor-relatable evidence of it being better than traditional weight loss methods, such as exercise.

Is there any medical evidence to support its effectiveness?

Intermittent fasting has existed for a long time, and its effectiveness has been studied since then. But in the old days, a very small number of people (usually under 50) were taken as a sample size to experiment, collect data, and analyze. Even though the results favored the effects of intermittent fasting, it nevertheless cannot be used as a generalization.

These results indicate that intermittent fasting provides health benefits other weight loss; studies show that it may help to lower the risk of heart problems and type-2 diabetes in some individuals; however, more research is needed to confirm this.

To do that, large-scale studies are called for. Moreover, other studies have been conducted on animals like rats and monkeys. Some of the claims about the advantages and disadvantages of intermittent fasting are made based on research.

What about longevity?

Longevity is another promise of intermittent fasting because of which it has grown so popular with even well-known celebs incorporating it into their lifestyle. In theory, it does affect lifespan as it slows down the metabolism, repairs and recycles damaged cells. But it's just a claim with limited scientific backing.

Most research on the effects of intermittent fasting on longevityis done on rats. Some rats who were put on intermittent fasting have been reported live 83% longer, which would not be possible for humans. However, even the possibility of living 20% longer evidence would be more than enough to make intermittent fasting more appealing to the masses.

Are there any side effects?

Known long-term or short-term side effects of intermittent fasting are minor. They include headaches, irritation, and fatigue. However, don't stretch yourself too much, too soon. One may develop heartburn, dehydration, and ulcers during the initial days, but your body will adjust accordingly.

Who should not practice intermittent fasting?

Pregnant women, people suffering from eating disorders, people who are chronically stressed, people with injuries who are in the healing phase, and people suffering from life-threatening diseases should not practice intermittent fasting.

INTERMITTENT FASTING AND AUTOPHAGY

The weight-loss world has shifted from diet charts to fasting for long hours. Staying hungry for a long time is a great way to lose weight. This technique is called 'intermittent fasting'. And it works on the principle of autophagy.

Auto- self

Phage- eat

The word autophagy means when something eats itself. And that is exactly what triggers the reduction of body mass in humans. Your body stays in the growth mode when you eat regularly. It generates energy to do work by using food molecules. The cells store the extra energy inside them in the form of fat. The waste products that enter the cells in the body (due to internal and external factors) gather inside them. This affects your organs, tissues, and eventually, your health and weight too.

But when you stop eating and start fasting, your body starts looking for sources of energy. As a result, the fat stored in the cells is broken down, and energy is released from them. Therefore, autophagy is a process where the body cells destroy their damaged parts and proteins and then recycle them in order to build themselves.

You can also view autophagy as a process where the cells in the body burn away the toxins stored in them and then use the remains to make something new. Many tissues and organs start the process of autophagy when they are deprived of food.

But How Does Your Body Know When To Start The Process Of Autophagy?

A signal must be sent to the organs to start breaking down the cells to produce energy. This can be done in many ways. It is not just fasting that can start autophagy in your body. Here are some other ways of losing weight that you can opt for.

Exercise

The more stress you create in the muscles and cells of your body, the more strongly the cellular cleanup phase will be triggered. All the extensive forms of exercise, including jogging, sprinting, weight training and physical training, regulate autophagy by inducing stress in the body. When the body is highly worked up, it needs energy that it gains by burning up the cellular waste.

Cold Showers

Yes, cold showers can also invoke healthy autophagy inside you. Studies have shown that people who swim during the winter exhibit higher levels of cell repair and recycling. Therefore, taking cold showers regularly can help you lose weight and stay healthy.

Steam Bath

Subjecting yourself to high temperatures through saunas and steam baths generates heat stress inside you. This heat results in the destruction and recycling of cancerous as well as damaged cells.

A trip to a spa can be good for relaxing, rejuvenating, losing weight and staying preventing diseases. Besides, exposing yourself to strong heat also helps to cure depression by naturally releasing heat shock proteins.

Intermittent Fasting

There are indicators in your body that activate or cease certain processes. The hormonal levels are one of them. When you begin intermittent fasting, you deprive the cells of essential nutrients. This activates the hormone glucagon in the body. This hormone works in opposition to insulin. While insulin increases blood sugar levels, glucagon brings them down to maintain the balance. The two hormones are like the ends of a see-saw.

When you are fasting, insulin levels go down, and, as a result, glucagon levels go up. This rise triggers autophagy. Your body gets the message that it is time to break down the stored fats in the body cells increase the insulin levels again.

Antioxidants

Though antioxidants do not directly invoke the process of autophagy in your body, they have been known to indirectly work towards it. Foods rich in antioxidants support the process when you are fasting, which in turn ensures that you undergo a healthy and balanced autophagy process.

Is There Something That Can Stop Autophagy?

There are factors that can stop your autophagy process. The major one is the mTOR. It stops the autophagy in your body when there are enough nutrients in the cells. It is highly sensitive and eating as little as 50 calories can increase the level of mTOR.

If you consume fats, it might not raise your insulin levels, and it might keep the mTOR levels suppressed. But high amounts of ketones and fats would break your fast.

Here is a list of things that you can take to keep your insulin levels low and let your body continue the waste removal process of your cells.

- Green Tea
- Coconut Oil

- MCT Oil

- Ginger compounds

- Galangal

- Reishi mushroom extracts

- Black coffee

- Apple cider vinegar

All these items can help to boost autophagy in your body.

Is It Just For Weight Loss?

Absolutely not. When the cells renew themselves by burning up the waste inside them, they do more than decrease your weight. Clean and healthy cells decrease the risk of developing diseases. Many forms of cancer, neurodegenerative diseases like Alzheimer's and Parkinson's, and metabolic and autoimmune diseases can be prevented through autophagy.

It helps fight infectious diseases and regulates inflammation. It has also been associated with fighting depression and schizophrenia. Fasting-induced autophagy is very helpful in keeping you healthy and preventing medical conditions. It is always good to get rid of the waste around and inside you. A clean environment is healthy and keeps you from getting sick.

Here is a list of major benefits of autophagy, both inside and outside of a body cell.

- Increases metabolism

- Decreases oxidative stress

- Increases genomic stability that prevents cancer

- Eliminates waste from the body

- Increases neuroendocrine homeostasis

- Decreases inflammation

- Increases lifespan

- Eliminates aging cells

- Improves muscle performance

Does Autophagy Help Women? how?

The ghrelin or the hunger hormone increases more quickly in women than in men. Women start feeling hungry again quickly after having a meal. Their bodies start craving food much faster and, therefore, are under more stress to look for energy sources. The cleansing of their body cells makes them less immune to catching diseases and helps them to develop a stronger immune system.

Does Autophagy Have Anti-Aging Effects Too?

Consider a real-life example. Assume that you have two cars, X and Y. You are somehow biased towards car X, and so you take much better care of it. You wash it every day, get it serviced every few months, and refuel the tank. But car Y does not see many bright days. It is just a backup option for you for the days X is out for servicing or repairs. You do not get its tank refueled, it stays covered in dirt and has been for just one servicing in years.

Now, which car do you think would last longer? Obviously, car X. When you pay attention to health and get the repairs done on time, faults and damages do not pile up. Your car X would stay as good as new even after years of driving, but car Y would start causing trouble very soon.

The same thing happens with the cells in your body. When the non-functional components and cellular waste keeps sitting inside the cell, it degrades your health and makes you look older. But when they keep recycling and renewing, it shows on your skin. Rejuvenated and youthful cells make your skin softer and healthier.

Autophagy is like a cellular garbage disposal system. Newer cells wash away the dead and unhealthy ones. This leads to increased elimination of aging cells. Autophagy slows down the aging mechanism of your body that makes you look younger and healthier for a long time.

How Does Your Body Renew Itself Through Autophagy?

Small things matter, and when it comes to aging, small things are the only ones that matter. Cells are what keep you healthy and sick. They store energy, carry oxygen and do everything for your body. And they are the ones that keep you from aging on the inside and outside.

Let us understand how this works. The cells in your body are continuously at work, so they experience a lot of wear and tear. The over-used cells eventually stop working, thus becoming useless. When this happens, the production of new and healthy cells is also discouraged by the useless ones.

These used up cells are known as senescent cells. A senescent cell is a living cell, but its functioning does not contribute to maintaining person's health. And while they do not contribute to anything, they do not let new cells to get formed in the body either. Over the years, the senescent cells keep accumulating in the body. They perform just baseline functions, stop the creation of new cells and promote inflammation. The worst part for women is that they speed up the aging of the nearby cells.

Autophagy clears away the damaged cells, thus making way for the youthful cells to appear. You stay young, healthy and energetic for a long period. Therefore, working towards burning up the waste in your body cells is a great thing for you to do.

Developing healthy habits in your life is a good way to live. No one likes an untidy home; while a shining home with new furniture is loved by all, including the ones who live there. Autophagy is a way to throw away all the old things from home and make space for refreshing new things.

TECHNIQUES OF INTERMITTENT FASTING

The great thing about Intermittent Fasting is the number of methods that you can use. If one method does not match your body and lifestyle, you can very easily switch to another. Is one method making you feel weak and dizzy?Wait for a few days and start using another method.

Your chances of success will increase when your body adopts an IF method. Here are the 13 most popular ways of starting IF. Each of them answers the three basic questions: How is it done, what to eat and what not to eat.

5:2 Diet

This is currently the most popular IF method. It is also known as the fast diet and is easy to carry out. The 5:2 ratio means that you eat regularly for five days a week and fast for the other two.

You can choose on which five days you would like to eat regular food, and which two you will fast. For these two days of fasting, must to restrict your calorie intake to 500 per day (if you are a woman) or 600 per day (if you are a man).

Although there are no restrictions on what you should eat during the fasting days, you can opt for one of the meal patterns that people generally follow:

1. Having three small meals (breakfast, lunch, dinner)
2. Having two big meals (lunch, dinner)
3. Having a small breakfast and a late lunch.
4. Having one big meal the whole day.

The diet works on restricting the calorie intake, which helps to burn fat cells. This diet is highly popular among those who want to lose weight. Besides, calorie restrictions also help to reduce insulin levels in overweight or obese women, thus reducing the risk of type 2 diabetes.

Since the calorie intake is limited for two days, here is a list of foods that would be suitable for you.

- Sufficient portion of vegetables
- Yogurt
- Eggs
- Fish or meat
- Low-calorie soups
- Black coffee
- Tea

Talking about what you SHOULD NOT have while fasting, you should avoid high-calorie processed foods, refined carbohydrates (bread, pasta, rice) and excess fats (cooking oil, animal fat, cheese). Not just that, this diet does not mean that the five days of regular food can include unhealthy processed foods. You cannot expect to lose your excess weight if you do not have nutritious food on all seven days of the week.

Meal Plan

Breakfast

Day 1: Toast with cream cheese

Day 2: Baked beans with a tomato and mushroom omelet

Day 3 (fasting day): Toast with peanut butter

Day 4: Grilled sandwich

Day 5: Toasted bagel

Day 6 (fasting day): Porridge with fruit salad

Day 7: Omelet with spinach and a tomato

Lunch

Day 1: Avocado and egg salad with smoked salmon

Day 2: Chicken fajita and a banana

Day 3 (fasting day): Chickpeas with reserved Bolognese sauce

Day 4: Green salad

Day 5: Baked potato with beans and cheese

Day 6 (fasting day): Fresh soup

Day 7: Chicken jalfrezi and rice

Dinner

Day 1: Potato wedges and chicken fajitas

Day 2: Penne and parmesan seasoned with Bolognese sauce

Day 3 (fasting day): Chicken soup

Day 4: Potatoes with onion gravy

Day 5: Rice and chicken jalfrezi

Day 6 (fasting day): Cod fillet and broccoli

Day 7: Petit Pois and a lemon sole fillet

There are no set rules as to when you should have your meals. You would need to experiment and discover what works best for you.

16/8 Fasting

This is the second most adopted method of IF by women. The 16/8 intermittent fasting method is a time-restricted way of promoting weight loss. You eat in an 8-hour window in a day and fast for the remaining 16 hours. Let us be clearer about what this window can be and how you fast for those long 16 hours.

You can stop eating at 7 p.m., skip the morning breakfast and start again by 11 a.m. The 11-7 window is your time to eat.

Or, you can have breakfast and lunch and skip dinner.

Your meals should focus on high nutritional value. If you think you can eat burgers and pizzas during your eight-hour window, you would not achieve much from this diet. You can take unsweetened drinks like water, black coffee and tea during the fasting period.

Please remember that your body will need some time to adjust to the new routine. You are likely to feel dizzy and nauseated in the beginning for at least a week. You might experience binge-eating tendencies to give up and start eating. But, once your body accepts your eating pattern, this fasting method can work beautifully for you.

Meal Plan

<u>When you eat early during the day</u>

7 a.m.: Veggie scramble

11 a.m.: Almond butter and apple

3 a.m.: Veggie and chicken stir fry

Evening: Decaf tea

When you eat during the middle of the day

12 p.m.: Smoothie consisting of a banana and peanut butter

3 p.m.: Pistachios with avocado toast

5 p.m.: Almonds with dark chocolate covering

7 p.m.: Whole meat and pasta

When you eat late

Morning: Black tea

1 pm: Blackberry chia pudding

4 pm: Carrots and guacamole

9 pm: Vegetables, quinoa, and grilled salmon

Eat-Stop-Eat

This is also known as a 24-hour dieting method. This is a very simple way to lose weight and build muscle that was discovered by Brad Pilon in his graduate research on short-term fasting. He found that one could easily burn 1600 to 3200 calories within 24 hours of fasting.

If you opt for the eat-stop-eat method of IF, you fast for 24 hours once or twice a week. It does not always mean giving up food for an entire day. You can have your last meal of the day at 5 p.m. and start eating the next day at 5 p.m. This way you eat something on both days.

No food is off-limits when you are not fasting, though you cannot eat anything in those 24 hours and are restricted to just sugar-free drinks. This becomes easier because you only need to focus on not eating for one or two days in an entire week. You can be carefree on the other days. Having said that, it is best if you avoid binge eating after the day of your fast.

Alternate-Day Fasting (ADF)

This approach calls for fasting one day and eating normal foods on the next. It has proven to be a very efficient method for weight loss and to reduce the risk of heart diseases and type 2 diabetes. There can be two broad patterns that you may follow:

- You eat as usual today, and nothing tomorrow. All fasting days are food-free and only involve water and unsweetened drinks.

- If you take in 2000 calories on a non-fasting day, it must to be cut down to 500 calories (25%) on the next day. (Modified ADF)

You could begin with the modified ADF and slowly shift to the actual one as your body starts allowing you.

But remember, as with the other IF methods, it is advisable that you still refrain from eating processed and unhealthy foods during the non-fasting days.

The Warrior Diet

This method of weight loss can be understood by knowing how it got its name. Think about the warriors during historic times. They had to prepare for battle or fight during the day. They could only eat what they liked at night – the warrior diet.

You eat zero or small portions of high fiber foods for 20 hours in a day and consume a large meal in the remaining four. You can call it an approach where you under-eat for 20 hours and overeat for the other four. The best way to follow this diet is by fasting for the entire day and then have a big dinner at night.

Make sure that you take in all nutrients during that one fulfilling meal of the day. Your body is going to need high energy levels and growth hormones to survive throughout the day. The Warrior Diet has five major benefits:

1. Improves concentration

2. Burns fat

3. Boosts energy levels

4. Increases cell repair process

5. Reduces inflammation

Meal Plans

Meal 1: Salad consisting of tomato, lettuce, carrot, oil, and vinegar

Meal 2: Meat, rice, pasta, butter, and veggies

Meal 3: Dessert

Overnight Fasting

This intermittent fasting method is very similar to the 16/8 approach. It involves increasing the number of hours between the last meal of your day and the first meal of the next day. The longer the period, the bigger is the impact on your body.

You can start by keeping a gap of at least 12 hours which should not be difficult. Then, slowly you can increase it to 14 and then 16 hours. You can start seeing the results within a few weeks. As you continue, your body will craveless food and will have better metabolism.

OMAD: One Meal A Day

This fasting plan is actually a very challenging one for beginners. You can to eat for just one hour in the whole day and survive on drinks for the remaining 23 hours. You pass a whole day fasting and choose a 60-minute window to consume a large meal. Research has proved the OMAD technique to be very useful for weight loss and tackling other health issues.

The one hour you choose to eat properly can belong to a fixed four-hour window every day. You can drink calorie-free and unsweetened beverages like water, coffee, and tea during the 23 hours.

This diet is very strict, for the most part. But there are no limitations on the nutritional profile of that one big meal of the day. However, high-fat and low-nutrition foods will only worsen your condition throughout the day.

Remember that you are likely to face serious hunger, fatigue, mood swings, low energy levels, and strong cravings during this method of intermittent fasting. You will have to resist hunger cravings and perseverance to control yourself. It is always best to focus on work and distract your mind during such situations.

The common take away

Each one of the above intermittent fasting methods, though different in approach, boils down to a single conclusion – you must increase the nutritional profile of your diet and reduce the number of times you eat. Creating gaps between meals lets your body burn extra fat and stimulates your metabolism.

WHAT NOT TO EAT DURING INTERMITTENT FASTING

Trying to lose weight is a challenging task, especially when you are a woman. You might struggle with your diet plans and find that exercising is always an activity for another day. Intermittent fasting seems to be your way to go.

And while you may know what exactly you need to eat during your fasting and the non-fasting days, it is even more important to know what is off-limits.

Here are the items that you need to stay away from if you are on an intermittent fast.

Sugar

It has been known to cause inflammation of the body, headaches and low energy levels if taken more than a prescribed limit. Weight-loss diets do not permit any type of sugar, whether refined or added. They are a big NO for those who are hoping to lose some fat.

Chewing Gum

High calorie and added sugars are the reasons why gums should not be part of a fasting diet. You may think that chewing gum for a while could take the hungry feeling away. But that is not how it works. It would harm your progress and make you want food even more.

Bottled Beverages

Energy drinks, juices, smoothies, teas, and even bottled waterfall into the list of restricted items. Most of them contain added sugars and high calories.

Chips/ Fries

Fried foods have unhealthy fats, salt and a large many calories. They lack fiber and proteins which are needed the most when you are eating less than you used to.

White Bread

Avoidfoods that are high in carbohydrates and have a low nutritional profile. Your goal is to cut down on calories and burn the extra fat, all while staying healthy and active. Eating white bread will keep you from achieving that goal.

Chocolates/ Cakes

Cakes, pastries, cookies, and chocolates contain high amounts of sugar and calories; these desserts should never be eaten during your intermittent fasting days.

Beer

It has been noticed that beer and some other alcoholic drinks cause weight gain, especially in women. Beer, in particular, bloats your stomach when you are trying to get rid of it.

Ice Cream

This is a NO for your non-fasting days. It's unhealthy, loaded with sugar and has a huge number of calories. It is better to make some yourself homemade ice cream with healthy ingredients.

White Rice

Research has shown that white rice is closely associated with obesity in females. It contains minimal proteins and fat and no significant nutritional value.

Energy Bars

Yes, they do have all the right nutrients. They increase your energy levels but, they have high sugar content in them. They harm you as much as they benefit you. It is best to avoid them.

Processed Meat

If you are confused about what it means, some examples are bacon, jerky, hot dogs, salami, and ham. These types of meat are high in salt and low in nutrients. While you think they seem apt for a fasting diet, they are not.

Frozen Meals

The manufacturers add sodium, a natural preservative in frozen foods and meals. Sodium retainswater, causing bloating. Make fresh, home-cooked meals instead.

Diet Soda

Well, you already know that diet sodais a myth. Its sugar levels violate all codes of dieting and fasting. Studies have shown that people who drank diet soda regularly had three times more fat than their counterparts.

Canned Soup

This is processed unhealthy and contains sodium as a preservative. It increases your appetite and decreases your ability to sense that you are full. Canned soups might not be a very wise idea when you feel hungry during your non-fasting days of IF.

Pizzas/ Burgers

Is it really needed to mention why these are on the list? Nothing in pizzas and burgers will assist you in your weight loss, except for veggies. Their saturated fats are also harmful to your heart.

Fried Chicken

This might be heart-breaking for a lot of you. But fried chicken is also off- limits. It causes inflammation and falls under the category of processed and fried foods.

It becomes easier to stay on the right track when you have a list of dos and don'ts. Eating the right portions and nutrients is essential to get the desired results through intermittent fasting.

FOODS TO EAT DURING INTERMITTENT FASTING

Fasting becomes a synonym for going without food for many long hours. Intermittent fasting has gained popularity for going in the opposite direction. The various methods followed in IF do not limit the nutritional profile of the diet, they still help women to lose weight. Each day, more and more women are shifting to methods of intermittent fasting, due to the flexibility offers them.

You can comfortably choose your own days of fasting. You also get to choose your meal on the non-fasting days. You can eat regular food, with normal portions of all nutrients. However, if you really want to take a maximum advantage during this fasting, here is a list of the best foods to eat. Try rotating these meals options during your non-fasting days:

High Fiber-Foods

These include nuts, beans, fruits, vegetables, meat, fish, tofu, high-fiber gummies, and other protein-rich foods.

Water

It helps to curb hunger by sending a signal to your brain that your stomach is full. Drink sparkling water, if possible.

Unsweetened Beverages

Black coffee, black tea, cinnamon or licorice herbal tea- all have appetite- suppressing effects.

Avocado

Eating this high-calorie fruit during your weight loss program will keep you satiated for many hours and keep hunger away.

Probiotics

The irritating side-effects of fasting can be eliminated by eating probiotic-rich foods like kefir, kombucha, and kraut.

Berries

Strawberries and blueberries are great sources of Vitamin C and boost your immune system.

Eggs

Obviously! They are high in protein. Having an egg during breakfast keeps your stomach satisfied for many hours.

Whole-grains

Eating carbs may not be the way to go when on a diet, but hey! A woman has got to eat. Whole grains are high in fibers and protein content.

Lentils

Boil them, add some lemon juice and take it all in. Lentils are great for helping you to losing that extra weight.

Seitan

Also known as white meat, this plant-based protein also helps during an anti-aging fast.

Hummus

It is healthy, creamy, tasty, and an excellent source of protein. You can also add garlic and tahini to make it more effective.

Salmon

It is well known for its dietary and longevity benefits, but it is even more popular because it contains brain-boosting omega-3 fatty acids DHA and EPA.

Soybeans

For vegan women, who do not eat eggs and meat, soybeans are the perfect food for your weight loss regime. They are high in protein, promote anti-aging and inhibit UVB induced cell damage.

Multivitamins

If you lose your appetite during those rigorous fasting days, multivitamins keep your body full of energy and help fill the gaps.

Salads

The best meal during your non-fasting period is a salad of broccoli, cucumbers, lemon juice, corn, lettuce, low-calorie dressing, chicken, olives, and sprouts.

DRINKS TO HAVE AND AVOID WHILE INTERMITTENT FASTING

Intermittent fasting is not a diet; it is just a schedule for eating. You stick to a plan about when to eat and when not to. Thus, if you want to lose weight, all you need to do is eat at fixed times. Of course, avoiding processed and unhealthy foods is always better when you are trying to lose body fat. Let's look at what you should and should not be drinking.

There are beverages that you should and should not drink on your fasting days. Let us begin with the ones you can take.

Drinks You Can Consume While Intermittent Fasting

Water

This is the best choice for your fasting periods. Drink as much water as you can. It keeps you hydrated, curbs hunger, regulates your body temperature and regulates the digestive system. It also helps to flush out the body's waste and helps it to maintain the right blood pressure.

Water can be in any form - sparkling, mineral or sea salt. You can add some cucumber, mint or orange to the drinking water as well. But stay away from bottled and artificially sweetened water. They raise your insulin levels, thus taking away all the benefits of your fast. Water is your best friend on your IF days.

Black Coffee

Caffeine increases your metabolism and curbs your appetite, making weight loss easier. Make sure that your coffee is black- no milk, no sugar, no cream. It increases satiety so that you can fast for a longer period without feeling hungry.

But your coffee should be limited to just one or two cups a day. Higher doses can lead to weakness, anxiety and a jittery feeling. Since you would be drinking coffee on an empty stomach, it would enter your bloodstream much faster and would have stronger effects. Also, try avoiding it when just before sleeping.

Tea (Herbal, Black, Green)

Sugarless tea is another good drinking option for your weight loss program. It induces the satiation response in the brain, giving you the feeling of being full. Green tea, in particular, increases adrenaline in your blood that releases the stored fat in the cells to be used as energy sources.

The antioxidants present in tea fight free radicals in the body. Intermittent fasting becomes more effective with tea as it promotes gut health, probiotic balance, and detoxification of the cells. Tea is a healthy drink when consumed in the right quantity.

Lemon Water

Remember that we are not talking about lemonade here. Fasting is strictly a no-sugar diet, and you must avoid high calorie, sugar-loaded items. Just take some mineral water and add a slice or twist of lemon to it. The purpose of this dash of lemon is only to add a bit of flavor to the water so that is a bit more palatable.

Lemon water regulates the digestive system and helps flush out the accumulated waste inside the body. It is a great way to stay hydrated and feel satiated.

Apple Cider Vinegar

The acetic acid present in apple cider vinegar helps your body to absorb nutrients and balance blood sugar levels. It is good for those with insulin resistance.

Apple cider vinegar is free of calories, improves digestion and reduces cholesterol levels in the body. It helps curb your hunger by suppressing your appetite. You can decrease the fat in your body by taking just a tablespoon of it every day. You should always make sure to dilute it in water to prevent tooth enamel damage.

Broths

If you opt to fast for 24 hours or more, a bone or vegetable broth is highly recommended for you. Make sure you stay away from the canned ones since preservatives will harm your fasting effects. A home-made broth is the best way to achieve weight loss. It satisfies your hunger and makes you feel full.

With the positives come the negatives. There is a whole other list of drinks that you should keep away from when you are trying to lose weight through intermittent fasting methods.

Drinks to Avoid While Intermittent Fasting

Alcohol

Alcohol is a big no-no for your fasting diet. Beer, in particular, contains lots of sugar and fat that will hinder your weight loss progress. Drinking alcohol during fasting hours decreases insulin sensitivity and slows down the burning of fat.

The whole process of intermittent fasting is based on a simple idea. It uses your stored fat to produce energy. But your body starts using the energy gained from alcohol instead of burning your body fat for it. You can drink small quantities of vodka, wine or whiskey during your non-fasting period, but make sure that you do not combine it with meals.

Milk

Milk is a major source of carbohydrates, lactose, and fat for your body. This makes it a high calorie and high sugar item. If you are serious about losing weight, it would be best to avoid milk.

Yes, milk is an important entity that needs to enter into your system. But it is quite heavy too. You can wave goodbye to your fasting progress if you drink a glass of milk. If you must drink it, keep it for your non-fasting days. But even then, keep the consumption minimal.

Energy Drinks

No energy drink comes without added preservatives or artificial sweeteners. It is understandable to feel weak and flow on energy when you are not eating. But energy boosting drinks are not a solution for your intermittent fasting days.

These beverages contain caffeine that makes you feel rejuvenated and high on life again. But so does black coffee. Opt for black coffee instead of sugary drinks.

Diet Soda

There is no such thing as a diet soda. It contains sugar, and calories that spike your insulin levels. It creates havoc with your blood sugar levels. They will break your fast. Your body would no longer be burning the fat inside and would be relying on the energy provided by these drinks instead.

Packaged Juices

Not every healthy thing that sells is helpful for your weight loss. Boxed fruit juice can never be a part of a fasting diet. Its high sugar levels disrupt the whole fat burning process in the body by increasing insulin levels. Just drink a glass of fresh home-made juice during your non-fasting periods.

Intermittent fasting works for your weight loss only if you make it work. Patience, self-control, and perseverance are all needed to stay on a fixed meal schedule. And remember, water is your best friend throughout your weight loss program.

PRO Tip:

Intermittent fasting methods are mostly based on long hours of fasting and a small window where you can cat as you like. This triggers binge-eating tendencies; you are likely to eat more than you should. Always remember that you are focusing on your weight loss. Even during the non-fasting periods, eat healthy and nutritious food. Stay away from unhealthy and processed foods, which will send you back to square one.

MYTHS ABOUT INTERMITTENT FASTING

Many of us would like to lose weight, but we want to do it without compromising our health.

Many women are highly cautious when it comes to losing weight with the help of intermittent fasting. They want to lose 10 pounds, but they are afraid that intermittent fasting might make them sick.

In order to put you at ease, allow me to bust some common myths about intermittent fasting.

Intermittent fasting is unhealthy for the body.

This is one of the most popular myths. It is a common belief that going without food will make the body weak and this entire process is very unhealthy.

Perhaps this is because we have a traditional belief system. According to the basic rule of thumb, we believe that we must continually consume food in order to keep our body healthy and safe. We believe that generally, food should be consumed regularly as a set of three meals a day and that this will keep our metabolism healthy and strong.

However, this is not always true. In fact, our body is remarkably capable of adapting to different situations. Constant consumption of food is not the best way to stay healthy. Thus, it is recommended to consume food in intervals and put your body through a fasting process regularly.

This is how IF helps you to provide your body with a very subtle healing effect in addition to helping you to lose weight.

Intermittent fasting slows down your metabolism

A lot of people believe that IF slows down your body's metabolism, and this can be harmful. In addition, they also believe that fasting could impede their weight loss.

The main reason behind this is that we are made to believe that we need three square meals daily to keep our metabolism active. Each meal we consume is full of carbs and sugar and that is the primary source of energy for us. However, we end up consuming a lot more calories than required, and this is what is utilized by intermittent fasting.

Intermittent fasting works towards stabilizing our metabolism by triggering growth hormone levels within the body. But it is worth mentioning here that prolonged fasting periods can prove to be harmful toour metabolism.

Intermittent fasting causes nutrient deficiency

Another common myth about intermittent fasting is that it causes nutrient deficiency. However, the truth is that regulated fasting does not cause any sort of nutrient deficiency.

There are some other reasons why essential nutrients might be missing in the body. These include low stomach acid levels, nutrient-deficient diets, imbalance in the body's blood sugar content, or even chronic stress situations.

If you want to lose weight through intermittent fasting, all you must to do is monitor your diet regularly. For instance, you would need to drink more water to keep yourself hydrated all the time. This will help your body to replenish the lost nutrients. Or, you might need to consume pink salt.

When you are fasting intermittently, your body is adapting itself to become more nutrient efficient. In this way, intermittent fasting allows you to store the nutrients for future use. Controlled fasting could also help you to boost your body's metabolism.

Intermittent fasting causes muscle loss

A lot of fitness experts complain that intermittent fasting can cause severe muscle loss. Is that true? Well, one theory suggests that when the body is made to go through prolonged low-calorific fasting or diet period, it tends to make use of the muscle protein to maintain its energy levels.

However, this is unlikely to happen if you are monitoring intermittent fasting daily. Many studies have been conducted on this subject. These studies found that fasting on every alternate day for a period of 8 weeks helped individuals to lose approximately 12 lbs. on average. However, there was no evidence of heavy muscle-loss. So, it is actually possible to lose weight and fat without compromising losing muscle mass.

Intermittent fasting causes eating disorders

While many women engage in intermittent fasting to lose weight, many believe that this causes heavy eating disorders. However, intermittent fasting is a weight-loss strategy, and it helps the body adapt to changing dietary requirements. That is why regularly practicing intermittent fasting does not cause any dietary disorders.

Sugar imbalance is one of the primary causes of eating disorders. So, if the sugar levels can be maintained by alternate fasting periods, these eating habits are likely to change. Having said that, if you are already a victim of eating disorders, it would be best to not engage in intermittent fasting. A lot of weight loss practices depend on your ability to control your hunger pangs. Thus, intermittent fasting, coupled with some resilience,could cause dramatic weight loss.

Intermittent fasting is not good for people with diabetes.

People with diabetes are expected to be extremely careful about their food habits and diets. Many people suggest that fasting is not the wisest choice for people with diabetes. However, intermittent fasting aims to control the body's blood sugar levels, making it a very good option for people with diabetes.

Intermittent fasting or alternating fasting periods work towards stabilizing the insulin insensitivity in the body. We are capable of adapting to the change in food habits and thus are more resilient to insulin changes. The sharper is our insulin sensitivity, the less insulin production is required for the body. As a result,body inflammation decreases dramatically.

For people suffering from Type 1 diabetes issues, it would be best if they could fast for a maximum of 12 to 16 hours a day. This helps adjust the body's glucose levels and thus helps you stay fit.

MISTAKES TO AVOID WHILE INTERMITTENT FASTING

Intermittent fasting might sound like a simple concept, but with only one simple mistake, all your weight loss efforts can go down the drain. One reason why most women fail to attain their desired results is that they have trouble adjusting to the plan. This is because, for many women, intermittent fasting is vastly different from the diet that they have followed in the past.

Additionally, you might be making a few mistakes which make the transition tougher. Let's look at some mistakes which must be avoided at all costs:

Thinking that it's a diet plan

Often, women tend to believe that intermittent fasting is a diet plan or a special form of dieting. Thus, they read articles and seek help/guidance about what to eat during, before and after intermittent fasting.

But this ancient practice isn't a diet -- it's simply a conscious decision to skip eating for a certain period of time. So, there's absolutely nothing you can eat during that time, and what to eat and what not to eat before/after the each fast varies from person to person.

Not choosing the right type of IF

Intermittent fasting doesn't refer to a single method; there are several. One is the 5:2 fast, where a person consumes a normal number of calories for five days and restricts their diet to less than half that number of calories for two days.

Then there is 24-hour IF, time-restrictive IF (where you eat only between four and five hours a day and fast for the rest of the day), and alternate-day IF. You should choose the one that fits your goals, schedule, and comfort level.

Too fast, too soon

When you practice intermittent fasting, you distance yourself from your normal way of living and eating. This puts some stress on your mental and physical health. Then there's the risk of procrastination and quitting too soon.

If you're a woman who snacks every two hours, then putting yourself into a hard-core straight 16 or 20-hour fasting routine might not turn out well. But your chances of success with IF will increase significantly if you start with seven to eight hours of fasting.

Over-stretching fasting time

The importance of starting out low was explained in the previous point. But it's also important to pace your fasting time period. For example, if you're starting out fasting for eight hours, then your next milestone should be as near to the 8 hours as possible. So, 10 or 12 hours is a better milestone than 15 hours.

Not adjusting with lifestyle

Intermittent fasting is like a ritual, and there are many factors in your everyday life which can influence it -- one of them being the lifestyle you lead. You will set yourself up for misery if you deliberately sign up for that something you know will clash with your fasting activity.

For example, if you're a gym- goer and train heavily for two to three hours, then if you follow it up with a 16 hour fast, it's prone to give health complications. Similarly, if you're going out or have birthday plans during the week, you should plan your IF to avoid clashing with these plans.

Consuming a high amount of carbs daily

Carbs are one of the major sources of energy for your body and the amount and type of carbs you consume determines your body glucose level. When you eat lots of carbs, especially processed ones, on a regular or daily basis, then your blood glucose level tends to reach a higher level.

But when you fast the other day for 10-12 hours straight, then there's a significant drop in your glucose level which can put major strains on your brain and nervous system. This can also make you feel grouchy, irritable, or moody. It is thus advised to eat less carb-based food and consume more vegetables and fats instead.

Binge eating

When you fast for 16 hours straight, its human nature to devour on whatever your eyes see first. But if you're practicing intermittent fasting for the sole purpose of losing weight, then you should closely monitor your food consumption after fasting.

IF works by using up the extra fat stored in your body as energy. Now, if you replenish that with consuming more calories than you lost, then your entire IF will be considered a failure. As a rule of thumb, don't rush to KFC or McDonalds to break your fasting. But you can have lots of fruits, vegetables, complex carbs, and mildly processed food.

Not eating enough

A complete counterintuitive to the previous point, one of the mistakes women make is they don't eat enough after their fasting hours. The main job of intermittent fasting is to use up the excess energy that's stored in the fat cells, not to deprive you of essential nutrients.

Additionally, when you don't eat for an extended period of time, you actually lose hunger and become less hungry (this is your body's way of fighting back). This is why some people tend to under-eat while some overeat. Thus, after your IF routine, make sure to refuel yourself with nutritious food like fruits, nuts, and vegetables - not with junk food.

Eating without realizing it

When you're on IF, to get the best results out of it, you should strictly restrict yourself from consuming anything, water being an exception. Beverages like coffee and diet soda can increase appetite which can make it difficult for you to continue with your fasting.

Not drinking (enough) water

While consuming calories or drinking any form of beverages is prohibited, drinking water is encouraged since it has no calories. As you're aware, the stomach releases an acid that aids in the digestion of our food.

When you're fasting, your stomach remains empty for a long period of time, which can cause acid to develop and accumulate. Accumulation of large amounts of these acids can cause stomach complications and irritations. Water prevents this situation by diluting the acid, thus keeping you focused on your intermittent fasting.

Not caring about the eating window

If you're fasting for long hours like 16, 20 or more hours, then you should include an eating window where you could gobble up some snacks or drinks. Fasting for such long hours could leave you too weak.

But having an eating window is not enough. You need to be careful about what you eat during this time. Keep the window short, for example, five minutes. Have some crackers, fruits, sandwiches, or a cup of coffee.

Eliminating exercise completely

While fasting, it's imperative to think that exercising is useless since you're not eating anything and the body is not getting the energy it needs to help you do your workout. But an average person has enough energy stored in the body to get you through your workout routine without feeling exhausted.

While you can't perform your usual drill session (if it's heavy), you can definitely do low-impact exercises like walking, cycling, or jogging. It will keep your body's metabolism going, taking you faster towards your goals.

For example, if you're planning to fast overnight, then you can hit the gym in the morning and have your protein shakes to build up muscles.

Not listening to your body

It's a fact that we all are different biologically. So we cannot have one single rule that is meant to follow by everyone on this planet. The online information about intermittent fasting is very general. To get the most out of your intermittent fasting, you tailor it to your own requirements.

For example, your stomach might start acting up after fasting for 4 to 5 hours. Now, as a rule of IF, you cannot eat anything during the fasting window. But if you continue following this rule, then chances are you'll develop some medical complications.

Therefore, you'd require an IF plan specific to your body. If you're having some problems when you're fasting, it's best to consult with a doctor.

Sitting idle

One of the biggest mistakes beginners do is sit idle while they're on fasting. When you're hungry and your stomach is crying for some food, it's natural to think about food and your cravings. You'll also start planning your post fasting meal. But this can become the biggest distraction and may even cause you to give up and break your IF.

So instead of sitting alone doing nothing, it's better to get engaged with something. You can spend some time on your office work, maybe learn a new skill online, watch a movie or play games. This doesn't be done indoors. You can go to the shopping malls, get a massage, watch a live football match -- it can be any type of activity. You stay busy in numerous ways.

Not persisting with it

Finally, women who start intermittent fasting give up to soon or after few months stating that it's not for them, it doesn't work, or they simply cannot do it. Barring any medical complications, you must push yourself through the fasting hours and stick with it to realize the amazing benefits of this technique.

You've to give it at least one and a half to two months to see some significant results. The points mentioned above will keep you on track with your intermittent fasting.

TIPS AND TRICKS FOR SUCCESSFUL INTERMITTENT FASTING

Things become much easier when you have special tips and tricks to accomplish a task. Intermittent fasting is no exception.

Based on the experience, here are a few tips and tricks that will help you out when it comes to losing weight with the help of intermittent fasting:

Identify your goals

This is the first step involved in any practice of intermittent fasting. You must first determine your goal. If weight loss is your primary goal, it is essential to have specific deadlines to reach that goal.

For instance, your goal could be to lose a few pounds in two, six, or ten weeks. This number helps you decide on the right intermittent fasting methods. It would also provide you with a deeper insight into the number of calories that you must lose and the number of nutrients that you must consume.

Determine the caloric needs

Intermittent fasting is useless unless you have a set plan regarding the caloric needs of the body. Essentially, there are no dietary restrictions when it comes to this eating habit. However, if weight loss is the priority for you, then you' should be able to create a calorie deficit in the body.

There are multiple ways in which you could determine how many calories you are expected to lose. You could also consider talking to a fitness expert for a deeper insight.

Pick the right method for intermittent fasting

This process has several different approaches. You could fast on alternate days or you could fast for certain hours during the same day. There are mainly four different methods you could use to practice intermittent fasting.

You should choose one type at the beginning of the regime and follow it right through. Changing your fasting method could prove to be really harmful to your body. Some of these methods include:

Eat Stop Eat diet: This is one of the primary methods of intermittent fasting. Using this technique, you should be able to fast for two 24-hour periods in a week. When you start your fast and when you end your fast it is not important. What matters is that you conduct the fast for a complete 24-hour period on two non-consecutive days. This is ideal for people who have had a taste of fasting before this. This is because if you are new to fasting, you might be prone to feel too hungry or eat too much as a result.

Warrior diet: This is another, much more comfortable diet that fasting enthusiasts might consider. Using this method, the individual eats less for a period of 20 hours during the day. That means, in a 24-hour timeline, the person consumes most of his calorie intake in the remaining four hours. For the rest of the day, they consume relatively less food. This is good if you want to lose weight drastically.

Leangains: This is a much more relaxed method of intermittent fasting. Using this method, the individual is expected to fast for much shorter periods of time and thus, it is a good option for people who have not tried fasting in the past. By utilizing this process, women looking for weight loss opportunities should be able to fast for 14 hours during the day. For the remaining 10 hours, they will be able to get all the caloric intake required for the body. In that 14-hour fasting period, the concerned individual should not consume any food but should focus more on low-calorie beverages for best results.

Alternate day fasting: This is one of the most popular methods for intermittent fasting. How does this work? For women seeking to lose weight, all you must do is consume 500-600 calories on two non-consecutive days each week. This sets you up for intermittent fasting and its benefits. If you are to do it more strictly, adding a third day of fasting becomes a rather interesting idea. Gradually, this process manages to create a calorie deficit in the body.

Keep yourself hydrated

If you are practicing intermittent fasting, always keep yourself hydrated by drinking a lot of water each day.

Some days, you might be fasting for the entire 24-hour period; some days you might be fasting for only 14 hours. Regardless, drinking sufficient water each day can help your body adapt to the fasting process.

Plan your meals in advance

Just practicing the usual intermittent fasting methods is not enough to lose weight. Before you jump into IF, it is essential that you prepare a weekly meal-plan.

This does not mean that you impose heavy restrictions on your diet all the time. This requires you to your calorie intake so that you make the wisest food choices while you are fasting.

Stay flexible.

When you start with intermittent fasting, it is entirely possible to go overboard first and to be too hard on yourself. But this could harm you a lot more than usual. The idea is to stay flexible with your diet plans.

Start slow, and if you notice changes in your body that suggest that it is not being able to adapt to the fasting methods, it would be best to change your plan and fast accordingly. That is why, it is imperative that you remain flexible with your dietary restrictions, and give your body enough time to adjust to the changing eating patterns.

HACKS TO SUCCESS: MY TIPS FOR SUCCESS WITH IF

There are many principal tips and tricks that I use till this day to continue to ensure my success. While intermittent fasting is all about the timing of your meals and fasting, it can be so much more if you decide to use all the resources available to you to keep it exciting, continue to learn new things, be creative, be consistent and prepare and be always prepared. Intermittent fasting along with the hacks discussed below will change your weight and your life forever.

Sharing is Caring

I am not certain if this will help anyone other than myself or not, but it did help and is still helping me. I have learned that I am best at all things in life when I am helping others along the way. I have always shared my knowledge with people day in and day and have become a coach of intermittent fasting to many. By encouraging others, I have simultaneously helped myself, because it's a shame to teach what you can't follow right? I won't be that type of coach. I practice what I am teaching. Me writing this book has helped me learn that I know so much about this topic, which is why I have been so much more successful this time around.

Apps to Download

Pinterest is such a good resource to use when it comes to planning meals to keep eating the healthier way. This app includes links to recipes, grocery lists, meal ideas, how to prep these meals, and more. YouTube, of course, is a great resource to review other people's struggles, peaks, and pits, before and after pictures, to hear their stories, to help you stay motivated and understand that most of what you go through while attempting to make this a habit, others have gone through the same things. MyFitnessPal's blog and community sections of its app is another great resource to use to join communities that are specific to intermittent fasting and all its components

These are good apps to have downloaded on your mobile device, iPad, or tablet. Using all your free time on these apps should be your new hobby instead of scrolling on your social media, especially since everything you see and hear will contribute to the success of making intermittent fasting a hobby.

Food Delivery Services

Some people decide that Meal Planning and Meal Prep is just not a realistic lifestyle for them. They may live a busier life than average, have a big active family, hate to cook, can't cook, don't want to cook, hate shopping, not creative, and more reasons. These people may choose to use a meal planning/prep or food delivery service to assist them with their meals.

Sometimes this can be costly, sometimes it may be affordable, but what it is, is convenient and by using this service you are still preparing in advance for what life throws at you during this change. You are still choosing healthier options, and being creative in what you eat.

Journaling

This lifestyle change will change your life forever. One day you will have changed so much that you may want to share your journey with others. If you decide to share, what better way to share than to go back and see how you felt each day or a few days. It is best practice to journal while you go through this journey. Journaling can be helpful in discovering what your negative triggers are, tracking your weight and measurement progress, tracking your feelings towards food, tracking your growth toward meal planning and food shopping and eating out and chosen food options, tracking your every step along the way. Your first journal entry should note why you are doing IF and explain your goals.

Sometimes people go as far as to go back to school for nutrition, or to be a trainer, life coach, and more, this journal will only assist you in tracking it all in real time. Your journal could be the road to success for someone or some other people who feel as though you once felt. This can also help you when you have those hard days and want to give up. Journaling can only help you on this journey; it is best practice for success.

Family Lifestyle Change

I wouldn't recommend making a drastic change, but after a few days maybe a week it's a good idea to start your family and sometimes even the company you keep around you to start eating what you eat and when you eat. If you are the cook and shopper in your house, this will be a better use of your time. You will only have to meal plan once, shop once, and cook a few meals that will feed everyone for a couple of days. Hopefully, this gives you more time during the week to add in exercise if you don't, or if you do maybe a second workout, or maybe give you a few hours of time each day to do something else you have been wanting to do, like maybe writing a book.

Brush your Teeth Earlier

Everyone should brush their teeth before bed each night. With intermittent fasting, it's better to practice brushing your teeth after your last meal. The taste of toothpaste and/or Listerine should keep you from wanting to do any further eating. This is just a mind trick, but it has been a successful, helpful trick that I still use.

How to Order at Restaurants

Know the menu before you go. I repeat, know the menu before you go. Most restaurants, even fast-food restaurants, have websites in which you can view their menu options. If you know what's on the menu before you go, you can be proactive in deciding what you will order as the best option for you. Have a few staple times that most restaurants offer: grilled salmon, chicken breast, shrimp, any seafood, fried chicken wings no breading or sauce, burgers wrapped in lettuce, salads, and more.

Most restaurants DO NOT serve appropriate portions of food. This is an advertising mechanism for the restaurants; it is an effective way for them to get you to continually come back and spend money with them. I mean, who wants to go to a restaurant that serves those small plate options? Most restaurants serve 2 and sometimes 3 times the portion that a person should be eating in one sitting.

To ensure you spend your money wisely but getting the food you pay for, while simultaneously ensuring that you are using good portion control, when you order at a restaurant it is good practice to go ahead and ask for a to-go plate and when your food arrives, split your food up by keeping an appropriate portion to eat now and package away the other 2 or 3 servings for later options.

Lunch Bag Prep

Every evening after dinner, clean the kitchen and prepare for the next day. This includes preparing my lunch bag for the next day. I add the following to my lunch bag each day. 2 full meals, 3-4 snacks, and 2-3 bottles of water and sparkling water. Although most days, I eat dinner at home, what if I didn't make it home in time to eat dinner, or what if football practice goes long, what if traffic is a mess due to an accident, what if I must work late, what if, what if, what if. Always be prepared and you will be successful. I have had unplanned events, which have forced me to eat in the car, and sometimes dinner is a few healthy snacks because I didn't have my meal with me. Be prepared.

How to Deal with Unplanned Events

Although unplanned life events occur, sometimes 3-4 times a week, as an intermittent faster, you still need to have a plan for the unplanned. Always have that lunch box/bag with you as previously mentioned. Know a few staple food options that are your go-to food options when you are on the go and don't have your own available food options. Think before you eat always.

Peer pressure is real, especially at social events, be sure to have a serious conversation with family and friends so they know you are serious and that they should not offer you items when it is not your feeding window and that your new lifestyle is not a joking matter and that you would appreciate they take it as an important part of your life. Make good decisions and be proud of those decisions that you make. Every now and then, I change my feeding windows for social events. I sometimes fast longer so that I can push my feeding window back to be able to attend social events and have dinner and drinks with family and friends.

Buy in Bulk

You may be thinking how is buying in buck related to intermittent fasting. It is vital for beginners and sometimes long-time intermittent fasters to always have food on hand to accommodate any cravings and their feeding windows. It is best practice to buy favorite snack foods in bulk if available. When you buy these items in bulk you can then use small ziplock and/or sandwich bags to create your own individual serving size (according to the food label) baggies to keep in your car, purse, backpack, at school, at work, in your gym bag, in your lunch box or bag, and more.

It saves you money buying in bulk than to buy individual items already prepackage, companies charge more for convenience, so when you buy prepackaged small cute individually packaged items, it costs more than buying in bulk and doing this yourself. This also ensures that you are only having a serving or 2 according to the food label. This also saves you from not being prepared and eating unplanned food items.

Consistent Routine

Appetite is trainable because it is driven by routine. Our bodies know and learn our routines, we are usually hungry when we expect to be hungry, not necessarily when we are physically hunger, again it could be that we are bored or need fluids. Practice makes perfect, right? Fasting is a skill that with intermittent fasting, you are trying to advance this skill.

Best practice would be at least start with a good routined new life as you endure this lifestyle change. That means to set your alarm and wake to start most days at the same time, specifically during the week to start. Eat your first meal and the second meal at the same times; you can have your snacks at whatever time during the feeding window. It is also best practice to workout at the same time of the day most days and take measurements, pictures, and weigh yourself on these same days. Meal plan the week before you will shop and cook the meals. Then shop on the same day, and cook and prep the meals on the same day so you start the week always with good habits.

Setbacks

Setbacks are sometimes inevitable when it comes to any type of life change; intermittent fasting is no different. Setbacks can include general fasting knowledge, lack of discipline, willpower, self-control, fear of missing out, lack of planning or procrastination, illnesses, that may or may not include medications, that prevent this type of fasting, lack of motivation, resistance to change, YOU, and much more.

YOU

You will be your biggest setback, challenge, and critic during this attempt to change. Many people have issues with confidence, self-esteem, feeling deserving, discipline, consistency, peer pressure, unawareness, and more, which ALL can contribute to YOU being your worst nightmare during this change and ultimately maybe your demise in many aspects of life.

You must realize you are the only person who can make a change in your life, and that goes for all the changes you want to make. You are responsible for your own happiness and if changing your eating lifestyle is what will make you happier, then this information gives you the knowledge to be able to make this change without help from anyone else. You can make this change happen for YOU, and only you. You should be beginning this journal to please only you and not just for appearance purposes, but for through and through happiness and well-being.

You must believe in yourself. You must know that you are your #1 priority and must be your biggest supporter. If no one else cares, you must care enough to change your habits and be consistent in the changes you decide to make. No one should be able to derail you from making such an important change in your life.

You are responsible for your choices. This is a lifestyle change, so if you mess up, just do better the next time, don't quit on yourself. Don't make decisions based on temporary needs or feelings; think about what you do as you do it to make decisions that are better for you overall in the future. Think about your future, do you want to be trying another diet in another 30 days? Do you still want to be in the same body with the same health in 30 days? Would you rather feel comfortable in your clothes and skin and feel healthy throughout?

Practice Makes Perfect

Getting acquainted with the process of fasting in general and testing your chosen time frames for your feeding and fasting windows can be a difficult time if you are used to eating many meals/snacks daily. Being motivated to continue to develop in this change is just as important as anything else that comes along with this change. Live each day separately, as in if something did not go to your liking one day, change your process the next until you have feeding and fasting windows that work well with your daily routine schedule. Mind over matter, you matter, so make sure your mind continues to know this fact to ensure you aren't resistant to this change.

Don't be Weak

During the initial change stage, there must be an increased amount of willpower, discipline, and self-control. You will be required to practice your self-control around others who are NOT on an intermittent fasting lifestyle. You need to have the willpower to refrain from ingesting calories during their fasting window. You need to have the discipline to create these time frames and stick to them, and when the feeding and/or fasting windows are broken, create consequences for yourself to ensure it does not happen again until it does not happen anymore.

Fear of Missing Out (FOMO)

Because of how you are used to living your life, sometimes you may feel like you are missing out on the fun surrounding social and/or family eating events, but consider the fact that you are making this change to perfect how you feel and how you look to ensure you are around for a long life to enjoy life. Family and friends may not be on this lifestyle and either will or will not support this change. Alcohol should be consumed in moderation. If you choose to drink alcohol, two or less daily drinks should be the max. Choose non-sugary spirits and alcohol volume dry wines to ensure you are getting the best buzz for your choice.

Holidays will more than likely be the biggest change for you and the biggest day to test you when new to this lifestyle. Holidays are all about eating and tasting everything with family and friends and making memories. Try to prepare in advance by either assisting with cooking to ensure meals are ready before/during your feeding window and choose your favorites to ensure you are satisfied and not as vulnerable after your feeding window closes. The holidays will test you.

Prepare, Don't Procrastinate

Preparation is key. Now that you have decided on your feeding window, ALWAYS, make sure you have your meals/snacks readily available during these times. Stay ahead of your schedule a day or so, to ensure you pack your meals/snacks if you are away from home when it is time to eat those meals/snacks to ensure. Even if you plan to be home, always make sure you take at least a few snack options with your wherever you go, by preparing in this way you ensure not to ever get caught out and about for hours with nothing to eat just wasting your feeding window away.

Not Reading Labels and Controlling Portions

Although your calories are NOT restricted when intermittent fasting, eating too much of even healthy foods can lead to weight gain no matter the type of diet/lifestyle you are following. To prevent this type of setback meal plan, use portion control, be consistent with choosing the most nutritious food choices, and measure your foods to ensure you are not eating too many servings in one meal.

Nonsense from Others

There are times in life when it's better to keep your goals to yourself. Keep your goals away from negative people, specifically keep negative people away from your goals and out of your life. To be successful in many things in life, you need a support system, which does not include negative people. You need someone who can cheer you on, someone who can motivate you, someone, who may be willing to join you, someone who doesn't add to your problems by persuading you to do what is against your goals. If you have these types of people in your life, do not tell them your plan of intermittent fasting.

Many people have their own preconceived assumptions about fasting, and intermittent fasting, and usually their views are without researched knowledge and education. It is important that you understand and know myth versus facts when it comes to intermittent fasting. People who have tried all types of diets seem to think they know them all, and they are very discouraging at times. During a lifestyle change as intermittent fasting, it is very easy to get discouraged, so stay the course and keep those people away, while you try this out yourself based on your researched facts.

WHO CAN DO INTERMITTENT FASTING AND WHO CANNOT?

By now, it should be clear that intermittent fasting isn't concerned with some religious beliefs or isn't done as a part of social or political propaganda. Intermittent fasting is a smart technique for losing weight.

However, even if you want badly to lose weight, intermittent fasting may not be your cup of tea. You heard that right! If it has to be practiced, it is better practiced rightly.

Fasting frequently is known to have ill health effects; however, intermittent fasting is in the news due to its health benefits and longevity of life that it provides. Some can do intermittent fasting and some cannot; here you can decide into which category you fall.

Intermittent fasting does not prove to be beneficial for everyone and can be detrimental for some people. So, here are a few of the cases in which you can practice intermittent fasting without any complications.

Who Can Do Intermittent Fasting?

- You are good to go if your body is used to dieting before; i.e. you have strictly monitored your calorie intake before.

- If you exercise, then your body can practice intermittent fasting.

- If you are single and do not possess any children, you can practice intermittent fasting.

- If you are in a relationship, your partner should be extremely supportive; if so, you can think of following IF

- If you are working, your job should be flexible,allowing for lower performance on certain days, usually at the beginning of the plan

- You can do it if you are a menopausal woman.

So, if you think your body is healthy enough and intermittent fasting can easily fit with the stream of your daily activities, it shouldn't be a bad idea for you.

But there is another side to the story. Here are few of the cases in which intermittent fasting is not recommended.

Who Cannot Do Intermittent Fasting?

- If you are married and have children, intermittent fasting may not be for you.

- If you are a professional sportsperson or an athlete, you might not be able to.

- If you have a performance-oriented job, you may not be able to.

In these situations, intermittent fasting will be a little difficult task for you. However, if you plan to proceed with caution so that it does not interfere with your performance at the job or your performance as an athlete, you can go try IF. In these conditions, intermittent fasting can be challenging, but not impossible.

Those who do intermittent fasting can also experience symptoms like sleepiness, anxiety, hormonal changes, etc. Also, women who perform IF experience far more issues than men. If you are male, intermittent fasting will be much easier for you.

WHO Intermittent Fasting is Not Recommended For

There are people who should never even think of following the intermittent fasting protocols. Some of such circumstances include

- If you are a pregnant woman, planning to be pregnant or are breastfeeding.

- If you have a history of disordered eating or are into disorderly eating.

- If your Body Mass Index (BMI) is below 18.5 or if you are underweight.

- If you are a Type 1 diabetes patient.

- If you are below 18 years of age.

- If you take a prescription for any medical condition, you should consult with your doctor before changing your diet or exercise plan.

- If you are chronically stressed and do not sleep well.

- If you have never tried dieting or exercising at all.

Intermittent fasting requires you to be disciplined and eat nutritionally, and if you have an eating disorder or have had one in the past, this may not work for you, and as well, create further health problems for you.

As mentioned above, fasting can interfere with hormonal growth; intermittent fasting should be strictly prohibited forchildren and teenagers as they are in a growth stage. If you don't want to stunt your natural growth, stay away from IF. Due to similar reasons, pregnant women should also not consider intermittent fasting.

In such cases, if you still want to lose weight, there are other morestraightforward options, such as monitoring your calorie intake, eating whole foods, drinking water and exercising a lot.

If you are thinking of following an intermittent fasting plan, you can now easily weigh your options and decide if you need to carry out the program or not.

DOES INTERMITTENT FASTING HAVE DIFFERENT EFFECTS ON MEN AND WOMEN?

In this day and age, push for gender equality is at its peak. Both male and female groups are advocating for it in many places ranging from sports arenas to the corporate world. However, there are fundamental biological, physiological, and psychological differences between men and women which cannot be denied.

New research is suggesting that the practice of intermittent fasting is having different effects on men than in women. And it seems that women are more susceptible to developing health complications or seeing no result out of it than men.

Why Fasting Can Be Harder for Women

The answer to this may boil down to hormones. Gonadotropin hormones released by gonadotropic cells are present in everyone. These hormones are responsible for the release of our sex hormones, progesterone from ovaries in females and testosterone from testes in males.

In females, the process seems to be more regulated. It's also more central to ovulation, which relies on cycles and schedules. Some theories suggest that when women fast or make changes to their habits and routines, their gonadotropin-releasing cells get more disrupted than those of men.

Furthermore, in the case of women, a type of protein known as kisspeptin is present in a higher concentration in their bodies. This causes greater sensitivity to fasting. This is one possible explanation as to why fasting is harder for women. In both males and females, fasting affects the nervous system too.

One research study pointed out that in the case of men, their nervous system became less agitated when they fasted, while in the case of women, the reverse happened, and their nervous system became stressed.

More research is required to conclude further on these subjects. There are some men who find it hard to fast while some women thrive on it.

The Case of Insulin Sensitivity

Insulin is the hormone present inside our body which helps in the breakdown and processing of carbs and glucose. It is secreted by the beta cells of pancreatic islets. When you fast for prolonged hours, there's no secretion of insulin, which means you get more sensitive to the effects of insulin, as they are present in such low concentrations. Some researchers in IF believe that this insulin sensitivity is required for weight loss and for IF to work.

But this works differently for men and women. As per a research study conducted in 2005, which involved eight men and eight women, it was found out that alternate day fasting adversely affected women and their glucose tolerance (which is associated with insulin sensitivity), while no or little effects were recorded on men. However, there have been studies conducted over the years which refute these findings. In some cases, they didn't find much difference between the sensitivity levels of men and women.

Fasting Effects on Autophagy

Autophagy is our body's mechanism that clears out dead cells and repairs damaged cells like mitochondria. The decrease in autophagy is linked with aging, while the increase in this process can slow down the ravages of aging. When we practice fasting, we affect our body's autophagy in some positive ways and is known as fasting-induced autophagy.

Just like glucose tolerance, there's very little research data in existence. However, one research study suggests that fasting doesn't have the same effects on autophagy in men as in women. In the case of men, the neurons present in the nervous system responded as we'd expect them to be, by undergoing the autophagy process, while in the case of females, the neurons responded by resisting autophagy. So, in the period of time, fewer cells were recycled, and fewer dead cells were cleared out in women.

This isn't necessarily a bad thing, and there's absolutely no research data that explains why IF works differently for men and women. This is just a proposed concept or theory.

How Fasting Affects Cholesterol Levels

Another study conducted and published in Clinical Nutrition ESPEN checked the changes in cholesterol levels before and after fasting. It noticed that women had lower levels of triglyceride and LDL when compared to men after fasting.

So, here women seem to have the upper hand. But more research is needed to conclude definitively.

Even if there are differences in results between men and women, they are not vast differences. And to reach a conclusion, researchers must conduct more studies, especially on a larger scale. But intermittent fasting is something which is recommended to both men and women. To get the best results, it is advised to seek advice from experts and doctors.

CAN INTERMITTENT FASTING EXTEND A WOMAN'S FERTILITY?

Fasting during pregnancy is not recommended. But to fast before getting pregnant and during the times while you are trying will be discussed here.

Getting pregnant and bringing a new life into this world is one of the most beautiful gifts that God has given to women. That is why women must be more cautious in ensuring the safety of their uteruses and reproductive systems when they decide to go on weight loss programs.

Extensive research is underway to determine whether fasting and dieting have a direct impact on a woman's reproductive system. With intermittent fasting getting trendier each day, more women want to know how it would affect their menstrual cycles and chances of getting pregnant. Some conclusions can be derived from the initial research, which shows that on some level, fasting and reproduction are linked.

Improvement in Fertility

Doctors who specialize in IVF treatments give a positive report about intermittent fasting. It has been noted that fasting has helped the couples who were struggling to conceive even through in vitro fertilization, or on synthetic contraception.

Whenever IVF specialized doctors find a patient who is struggling to conceive, the first thing they do is analyze their diet. The amount of nutrition and calories a person consumes affects their chances of getting pregnant. Some people are even asked to take up intermittent fasting to achieve an ideal body mass index.

Gynecologists have noticed that fasting has significant benefits in increasing a woman's fertility. This happens due to the many changes that her body goes through while fasting. Intermittent fasting plays a direct role in improving fertility by:

- Pulling out excess and synthetic hormones

- Cleansing the liver

- Alkalizing the bloodstream

- Rebooting the natural hormone process of the body

- Flushing out the unwanted toxins

- Helping women to attain the right BMI

- Decreasing inflammation

- Balancing blood sugar levels

- Boosting metabolism and immune system

- Getting the reproductive system ready

Extension in Fertility

Another important fact that has been noted is that intermittent fasting extends a woman's fertility. This allows older women to have kids during the later stages of life. Studies suggest that restrictions on food intake can help to replenish the depleted ovaries under the right conditions.

A study conducted on mice showed that when calorie restrictions are put on the adults, it disables the age-related decline in the quality and quantity of oocytes (egg precursor cells). It also increased the reproductive lifespan of those mice along with the chances of the offspring surviving after birth.

Multiple studies have indicated that manipulating nutrition and restricting calorie intake can have great effects on the underlying pathways in the human body. There have been discussions and theories about how female fertility can be put on hold for later stages without damaging the pathway to pregnancy.

The specifics are not very clear on the number of calories and nutrient intake that is appropriate to achieve this extension. Once the underlying molecules are found and scientists find a way to manipulate them, it would help in treating many fertility problems and even extend the female reproductive system.

Research is underway to find out how eggs begin to grow and how this process can be slowed down. This, in turn, would directly help in enhancing fertility.

Intermittent Fasting Effects in Women Over 50

Your body undergoes many changes once you turn 50. The major ones are lower metabolism, achy joints, areduction in muscle mass, and sleep issues. You no longer have the body of a youthful person. Some foods might not suit you anymore and some activities mightcauseyou pain. And it is this time when there is a high risk of developing diseases like diabetes, heart attacks, cancer, and other metabolic disorders.

Intermittent fasting is an excellent method to remain more youthful after you reach the age of50. The anti-aging benefits of IF help you stay young and prevent various age-related illnesses.

Belly Fat

The reason behind most diseases is the waste stored in the body in the form of excessive fats. The main principle behind IF is autophagy, in which cells destroy the non-functional components and fats stored in them to release energy. This cleanses the body and keeps you from getting sick.

Belly fat is one of the biggest concerns in women post-menopause. Fasting helps to reduce this belly fat, gets you in good shape, improves health. This reduces the risk of metabolic syndrome in women over the age of 50. For those who do not know about metabolic syndrome, it is a collection of health issues that increase the risk of heart diseases and diabetes in post-menopausal women.

Muscle & Joint Health

Studies have shown that periods of fasting produce a hormone in the body that affects bone minerals like calcium and phosphate. This increases your bone health and saves you from the risk of getting arthritis.

Also, calorie restrictions and the burning of fats have been associated with the improvement of muscle health in elderly women.

Cancer & Depression

Fasting inhibits the pathways that lead to cancer and slows down the growth of tumors in the body. Middle-aged women can fast for more extended periods to curb the risk of developing severe diseases.

Eating healthy food makes you feel better. Your body undergoes many hormonal changes when you restrict the intake of food. These help you control your mood swings and stay happier. Also, being in good shape and feeling active is a boost to your self-esteem. Research has shown that fasting can fight depression.

A Word of Caution

The post-menopausal period can be tough for many women. If you feel uncomfortable while fasting, it is best to consult a doctor and know which type of fasting is best for you.

INTERMITTENT FASTING FOR PREGNANT WOMEN

Intermittent fasting focuses on restricting the eating window to a limited number of hours and fasting during the rest of the day. It has helped a lot of women to lose weight, regulate digestion and boost metabolism.

But pregnancy is not the time that you need all these benefits. Losing weight is not something you should aspire to while a baby is growing inside you. That goal is for the time when your delivery is done, and you wish to come back to your pre-pregnancy body.

Pregnancy and Intermittent Fasting Do Not Mix

Most experts say that it is not a wise decision to fast during pregnancy, even if you are following IF. The main reason for this is how IF works in the first place. The basic principle behind the techniques relies on burning extra body fat leading to weight loss. But pregnant women are supposed to create and store fat for the baby instead of losing it.

Not just that, IF methods reduce the blood sugar levels in the body while trying to generate energy from the fat stored in the body. And low blood sugar is very bad for the fetus. This strong contradiction is why fasting and pregnancy do not go handinhand.

If you are already a strict follower of IF methods, you could consult your doctor about toning it down instead of giving it up completely. But to start while you are pregnant is not a good idea.

How Is the Unborn Baby Affected by IF?

If you opt for intermittent fasting during your pregnancy, you are preventing your body from getting enough protein, folic acid, vitamin B12, iron, vitamin D, calcium and all other vital nutrients needed for the baby to grow healthily. A mother's malnutrition directly affects both the child and the child's delivery.

Dieting behaviors during pregnancy have caused long-term defects and other consequences for both the babies and their mothers. For example, research showed that lower calorie intake during the three trimesters was directly linked to the students with lower math scores. There had been a lack of brain development during the first trimester of their births.

There Might Be Long-Term Outcomes

Research has shown that pregnant women who fast as a traditional or religious practice face long-term consequences.

There have been many cases where mothers who fasted during their expecting period gave birth to babies with certain fetal effects. These include:

- Low birth weight

- High birth weight

- Cognitive impairment

- Gestational diabetes

- Breathing problems

Though it is not a conclusive result, no mother would like to take this chance with her child. The health of the baby is always a greater priority than losing weight.

Fasting During the First Trimester

Your first trimester of pregnancy is a roller coaster ride for your stomach. You are simultaneously hungry and nauseous throughout the day. You may feel the need to eat all the time. But every time you do, you may feel like throwing up.

Carbohydrates do not give you a satiating feeling, and fat makes you throw up. You may find yourself struggling to decide whether you should eat. With this unsettled and unsatisfied stomach, you can hardly manage to follow the rules ofa fast.

The first three months of your pregnancy are crucial for the healthy development of your child. You must followa nutritional diet. You can eat 10 times a day as long as your body is accepting it. Therefore, this is not the time for you to even think about avoiding food and fasting.

Fasting During the Second Trimester

Nausea settles down quite a bit during the second trimester of pregnancy. Your body accepts food easily and the urge to eat all the time decreases a lot. But even then, you should always give priority to eating the important nutrients first.

Since you tend to feel full more often, it becomes essential to consume all relevant proteins, micronutrients, and calories before you reach satiety. Your second trimester would be virtually intermittent fasting only.

The best part is that your body throws into a pattern of mindful eating cues naturally, and you do not have to force it to follow a specific schedule of eating and fasting.

Fasting During the Third Trimester

This is the worst time to even think about getting into intermittent fasting. Your need for calorific and high-protein content is at its highest at this point. With the baby taking up so much room, it would be practically out of the question for you to eat large meals in one go. This means that even if you try fasting, your body will strongly resist it.

Insulin resistance and blood sugar levels are very high during the third trimester of pregnancy. You, therefore, would

need to split up your meals and snacks throughout the day.

Safe Fasting During Pregnancy

Continuous and rigorous fasting is not recommended for pregnant women. But you can still fast safely for a few days if you follow some simple tips.

- Keep yourself hydrated throughout the day. Drink lots of water and fresh juices so that you do not feel starved.

- When you eat during your non-fasting period, start with little quantities of light food. Eating heavy foods in large quantities is not good for your baby.

- Ensure that your food is high in nutritional value. You need to maintain your energy and nutrient levels during your pregnancy period.

- Rest and do not exert yourself by walking too much or working out when you are fasting. Save your energy for consumption and bodily functions.

- Stay away from drinks with high sugar and caffeine. Keep yourself calm and do not indulge in anything that causes stress.

Listen to Your Body

You eat for two when you are pregnant, and obviously you would wish your baby to be as healthy as possible. You are likely to gain weight since the weight of the baby would be added to yoursand because you would start eating more than usual.

Pregnancy is a period where you worry about your baby's health more than your own. It becomes necessary to eat healthy food with high nutritional value at regular intervals. The demands of the body are different, and cravings are stronger in moms-to-be. It becomes difficult to eat just for a few hours a day.

It is damaging to you and the baby to starve yourself when your body demands food. Your body gives you a lot of signals when you are pregnant. Listen to them, and focus on the health of the life growing inside you.

Warning Signs When Fasting

Do not continue your fast if you feel that your body is not accepting your fasting routine. Break your fast immediately and start eating regular portions of food with good nutritional value. Your body will show you signs when it is not able to manage your pregnancy and fasting together.

Some of these symptoms will include weight changes, less urination, dehydration, constipation, headache, weakness, nausea, vomiting, and even a decrease in baby's movements.

Is There Any Positive Side of IF During Pregnancy?

The advantages of intermittent fasting still stand strong. It increases your metabolism and burns excess fat. In some cases, intermittent fasting has even led to good pregnancies. You may be able to consume adequate nutrientsto have a perfectly healthy baby.

But that is a chance that a mother can avoid taking. Taking unnecessary risk during pregnancy is not recommended.

Talk to Your Doctor

You cannot possibly know everything about pregnancy, even if you are not a first-time mother. Your gynecologist is the best person to talk to whenever you feel uneasy or have some doubt about your bodily functions.

Never hesitate to call him/her or to make an appointment to clear up your doubts. Your baby might need some extra attention or medications for its growth and survival.

Giving birth to a child is the most beautiful experience in the life of every woman. There are many ways by which you can reduce your pregnancy weight after you have given birth. But if you stay focused on your weight throughout the nine months, your kid might have to face some serious issues later in life. Keep fasting for when it is safe. Focus on providing the best nutrition to your unborn baby.

INTERMITTENT FASTING COMPARED TO OTHER DIETS

One way to compare diets is in an apples-to-apples manner; let's make the USDA recommendation the benchmark. IF and other diets will be compared against it, and the advantages/disadvantages of each diet will become evident.

When comparing, we'll also discuss parameters like the convenience of following the diet, how it affects nutrition, the health benefits it provides, and weight loss promise.

Intermittent Fasting

- Ease and Convenience Level

There are many types of intermittent fasting. So, the convenience level will depend on which type you are on and your lifestyle. Many forms of IF give peoplethe flexibility to choose the one that's in line with their daily duties. This makes intermittent fasting highly flexible compared toother forms of restrictive dietary habits.

- Nutritional Benefits

If you're currently on any form of IF regime, chances are you won't be able to meet the nutritional guidelines of USDA on your fasting days. But the chances of reaching some of the guidelines on a weekly basis becomes much more possible if you handle your eating days the right way.

But whether you'll meet the recommendations will depend primarily on the type of IF you're practicing and the kinds of food you consume during the eating window. Let's break the nutrition into two types.

Calories

Most, if not all, people decide to embark on an intermittent fasting journey to reduce their calorie intake and get lean in the process. Now, one thing to remember is that each macronutrient is essential for the survival of human beings. So, the whole concept of any IF or other diet plan is to cut down the excessive intake of calories and not restrict it to zero. That would obviously be hazardous.

If you're following any of the intermittent fasting plans, chances are you'll meet the recommended calorie intake guideline. Most IF plans have an eating window during which one can consume food. For example, the 16:8 IF has an 8-hour eating window. Also, there are no restrictions on the types of food you can consume during that timeframe (except for junk foods, obviously). So, you can easily hit the recommended level by eating enough calorie-defined

meals.

But when you're following specific types of intermittent fasting, like the 5:2 one, where you consume food for five days and follow this up with heavily-restricted fasting for two days, you may not be able to meet that recommendation on those two days. This plan restricts your diet so much so that you may not even complete half of the quota. The solution? You consume more than the recommended level during your normal eating days to replenish the shortcomings and meet the weekly calorie recommendation.

Food Groups

Food groups are fruits, vegetables, grains, and dairy products. During fasting days, chances are you won't be able to meet the food group recommendations. For example, let's take the case of carbohydrates and the 5:2 IF. On this specific diet, women are restricted to 500 calories per day on their fasting days.

As per USDA recommendations, you should consume 130 grams of calories daily to maintain good health. But that would mean more than 500 calories per day, which would void the 5:2 IF rules. The same goes for other macro-nutrients like protein, vitamins, fats, etc.

To replenish this deficiency, you would have to consume enough of these food groups during the eating window on your eating days.

Health Benefits

IF has been shown to have many health benefits besides weight loss; some of these include improved brain and heart health, a lower risk of diabetes and blood pressure, cell recycling, and delayed aging.

Weight Loss Prospect

Most people on intermittent fasting have reported losinga considerable amount of weight within two to three months, which suggests that it is an excellent diettype for people looking to lose weight.

3-Day Military Diet

Like the 5:2 IF plan, the 3-day diet is a diet that requires you to limit your food intake for three days of a week. But unlike the 5:2 plan, the three days don't need to be consecutive ones; they can be spread across the week. People who follow this practice have only a limited number of foods they can eat during those three days.

Ease & Convenience Level

As the 3-day plan severely restricts your diet, you must be very diligent about what you eat. You must measure the calorie level of food and their constituents. This must be done for the entire duration of the program. Some people may find this inconvenient as three days is almost half of the week.

Nutritional Benefits

Severely limiting your food intake for three days will not enable you to get the required number of calories or food groups for the day. It's almost impossible to be on this diet plan and eat the recommended amount of fruits and vegetables. Eating for the rest of the four days may make up for weekly recommended intake.

Health Benefits

The 3-day diet only modifies your lifestyle for three days. Such diets have been shown to provide little health benefits. Moreover, they aren't sustainable. If you don't stick to specific days and go on and off, the effects may even become detrimental and increase the possibility of binge eating and other disorders.

Weight Loss Prospect

People do cut down some weight after following this diet plan, but the bad news is that it is most likely temporary. A three-day only modified diet is highly unlikely to reduce fat, especially when the other days are left unchecked. What we see as weight loss might be water weight loss. In this case, when you resume the eating pattern, you will regain weight naturally.

Body Reset Diet

As the name suggests, you reset your body and start with an unusual eating habit. When you get on this diet, you must spend the first days surviving only on smoothies and avoid any food in solid form. This diet was developed by Harley Pasternak, a reputed fitness trainer who has worked with celebs.

Ease & Convenience Level

The best thing about this diet is it lasts for only 15 days. So, anyone who wishes to do this won't have to compromise or adjust their lifestyle for long. The only thing to take care of is to follow the protocols of this program diligently to get anything out from it.

Nutritional Benefits

Your calorie intake will be much less while on this diet. In fact, in the initial five days, you'll consume less than 1,200 calories per day. But on the flip side, you'll consume enough fiber, carbs, fats, and protein during the period time, which makes this diet nutritionally great.

Health Benefits

Because of the short timeframe of the diet, you will not likely see any health benefits. But it may help to improve your health if you continue with the recommended diet plan for a few more months.

Weight Loss Prospect

When you're on a liquid diet, the chances are high that you'll lose some weight, especially if you're following a high-calorie diet. But when you lose weight too quickly, it becomes hard to maintain.

Fast Diet

A slight variation of the 5:2 intermittent fasting, in this program you restrict your calorie intake for two days of the week, but still follow a calorie-defined meal plan as opposed to a non-restrictive meal plan like 5:2 IF.

Ease & Convenience

It might seem too farfetched for some people because the eating days are restricted too, and you must consume enough food to keep you going throughout the day. The calorie intake will obviously be based on your day-to-day activities, but it restricts you from consuming anything extra. People following the 5:2 IF plan have no such restrictions and have foods of their choice.

Nutritional Benefits

From a nutritional point of view, it might be the best diet plan simply because only nutrient-dense and healthy foods make it into the menu. During your fasting days, you'd be restricted to 25% of your daily USDA calorie recommendation. So, on such days, it might be impossible to fulfill all your nutritional requirements.

Health Benefits

Some studies conducted have shown the same benefits as in the case of IF diets, but more research is needed to reach a conclusion.

Weight Loss Prospect

People on this diet plan do report weight loss, but its comparison to 5:2 IF, where there is no restriction of calorie intake during eating days, is ongoing. So, whether it is worthwhile for weight loss is still unclear.

Master Cleanse Lemonade Diet

With the alluring claim that you can lose 10 pounds within 20 days, the Master Cleanse Lemonade Diet has lemon at its core, which is a celebrated fruit around the world, specifically for weight loss. It also claims to cleanse your body from inside. You're put on a lemon-juice-only diet for at least 10 days, which is your only source of nutrients and calories.

Ease & Convenience

Even though it's simple, most people will have trouble switching to a lemon-only diet, even for a short period of time. So, it's not for everyone.

Nutritional Benefits

With a lemon-only diet, it won't be possible to meet any of your nutritional requirements. With this diet, where you'll consume 10 glasses of lemon water daily, along with sugar, you'll consume around 650 calories per day—less than the recommended level.

Health Benefits

With no supply of solid food, it's not likely to yield any health benefits. On the other side, some people may face health complications like dizziness and fatigue. Even though the diet claims to detox your body, more research is needed.

Weight Loss Prospect

When you consume nothing but lemon water for 20 days, it will naturally lead to weight loss. Whether someone will lose 20 pounds or not will vary from person to person. But the weight loss might not be sustainable once you return to normalcy. With binge eating, you may gain more weight than you lost.

SHOPPING LIST FOR YOU WHEN ON IF

Meat

Ground beef, sausages (chorizo and Italian), bacon and pork are best for intermittent fasting. They are excellent sources of protein, vitamins, and minerals. Red meat contains a lot of iron and is one of the main sources of vitamin B12. Women need to maintain a balanced diet, even while fasting.

Though it is a big part of a healthy diet, you must be careful with your hygiene while storing, preparing and cooking meat. Avoid meats that are high in fat. Choose the leanest meat that you can find at the store. Try buying unprocessed meat products. Salami, beef burgers, pâté, pies, and sausage rolls are processed meat items and are not very healthy.

Fish

Fish is a high-protein food that contains omega 3 fatty acids, or the "good" fats. These fats are very good for the heart, brain, and bones. Fish has been known to be helpful in prenatal and postnatal neurological development. Though you can complete the nutritional profile of your diet by taking fish oil supplements, eating fish directly always has more advantages.

Some of the fish that you can consume are the wild salmon, anchovies, sablefish, sardines, tuna, and Arctic char. They have lower environmental contaminants and are eco-friendly.

Chicken

It should not come as a surprise to you to know that chicken is a great addition to a weight-loss diet. The high protein content sustains your muscles. This low-fat food is healthy and full of minerals like calcium and phosphorus. Also, it drastically reduces the risk of getting arthritis by keeping your bones healthy.

Chicken helps reduce your stress. It also contains magnesium, which enables you to fight the symptoms of your PMS period. This makes it a very important item to put on your shopping list before those mood swings kick in.

Fats

Do not hesitate to add heavy cream, olive oil, coconut oil or butter to your list. Butter and cream are very satiating.

All these saturated fats are good for losing weight if consumed in normal quantities. All types of creams made from milk contain calcium, riboflavin, vitamin A and phosphorus. These nutrients should always be a part of a balanced diet.

There is another reason why these fats are a good option for your fasting diet. They make you feel full much more quickly than carbohydrates.

Dairy

Everyone knows that milk is good for the body. It helps in the growth of your bones and muscles. Drinking high-fat dairy products lower the risk of weight gain in the long run. Yogurt, low-fat milk, and ghee all help to reduce the risk of heart disease, type 2 diabetes, and high blood pressure levels.

The most important thing is that dairy products are high in nutrients and make you feel satiated quickly. Your calorie intake remains low, and you eat healthily.

Fruits

Fruits should also be part of a weight-loss diet. They are a ready-made pack of vitamins and fibers. This low-calorie food is recommended for those looking for losing weight. As added advantages, they lower your risk of diabetes, high blood pressure, cancer, and heart disease.

Some of the best fruits to eat during intermittent fasting are:

- Grapefruit

- Apple

- Berries

- Peaches

- Plums

- Passion fruit

- Rhubarb

- Kiwi

- Melon

- Orange

- Banana

- Avocado

These fruits help keep you satiated; fruit is an important part of a fasting diet. Do not forget to keep some fruit in your bag whenever you are out.

Vegetables

A trip to the grocery store should always mean vegetable shopping when you are trying to burn that extra fat. Veggies have a lot of fiber, vitamins, and minerals, which boost your metabolism and help you to lose weight. They are very good for your body and help to prevent diseases. Some of the most effective vegetables that must be on your shopping list are:

- Asparagus

- Spinach

- Lettuce

- Mushroom

- Cauliflower

- Broccoli

- Chili peppers

- Pumpkin

- Carrot

- Beans

- Jackfruit

- Spices

Believe it or not, spices help you to lose weight. Black pepper is the most effective of them all. It increases metabolism, regulates digestion and helps with cell health by destroying the fat in them. It is essential for the digestion of proteins and other solid food in the stomach.

Chili powder increases your body's fat-burning capacity by 25%. It also decreases the cholesterol levels in the body. Cayenne pepper has been known to decrease aperson's appetite, and hence their calorie intake. Hot sauces and spicy foods should be on your preferred list of foods while fasting.

Miscellaneous

Apart from these categories, there are some items that you should buy during your intermittent fasting days. Eggs are one of the important ones.

Make hard-boiled eggs or scrambled ones a part of your daily meal. They make a perfect meal to feel full without taking in fat.

Toasted bread and buns can also be a part of your meal. They are a good source of carbohydrates and have fewer calories. Pair them with chicken or hot dogs to make a delicious meal.

Beverages

When you are in your fasting period, drinks are what support you. Stay away from sweetened and processed drinks. You can have black coffee, green/black/herbal tea or lemon water when you feel hungry. Therefore, remember to put coffee, tea, and lemons on your list. Also, do not depend on bottled drinking water.

MEAL PLANS FOR IF

Intermittent fasting lets you eat whenever you want and however you want. If you are dedicated to losing weight, then you should follow a proper diet. Though fasting techniques will help you to lose fat, you can increase the rate by eating foods that regulate the burning of the extra fat in your body.

Even if you decide to follow a meal plan for your diet, you will still have many things to eat during your non-fasting period. Whether you are following the 16/8, 5:2, 24-hour or alternate day method of IF, there are still times when you can eat what you like. However, you will get the most benefits from your weight-loss regime if you stick to certain foods at your breakfast, lunch and dinner times. To help you make the right choices, here are the items which you should eat at these times.

Breakfast

If you are following a fasting plan that allows you to have an early breakfast, then you should try consuming these foods.

Green Smoothie

The low sugar levels and healthy fats in it keep you satiated until lunch, and it is great for regulating digestion.

Preparation Method

Add avocado, chia seeds, coconut milk, and spinach to your blender and drink it up.

Mint Chip Protein Shake

It is full of protein, greens and wholesome ingredients.

Preparation Method

You just need to mix avocado, Greek yogurt, protein powder, mint/peppermint, milk, and spinach.

Egg Muffins

Eggs are a great source of proteins and important vitamins.

Preparation Method

All you would need for making delicious egg muffins are bell pepper, onions, tomatoes, eggs, some spinach, salt, and hot sauce.

Chocolate Coconut Protein Balls

These proteinballs are satiating and keep you full for a long time.

Preparation Method

Mix coconut, oats, chocolate chips, honey, and some protein powder, and your healthy breakfast item is ready.

Oatmeal

The traditional breakfast for dieting people is oatmeal.

Preparation Method

Choose your flavor and just add some milk.

Hard-boiled or Scrambled Egg

The goodness of eggs is known by all. The vitamins and other nutrients present in an egg are good for your bones and muscles.

Lunch

This would be included in almost all meals during your fasting and non-fasting periods. Make it a nutritious meal with moderate calories and high satiation. The following items can help you achieve that.

Baked Potato

They give you steady energy and lasting fullness for a longer period. They are very high in carbohydrates, vitamins, and fibers.

Roasted Vegetables

Veggies are a ready-made source of all the nutrients that your body needs. A high amount of vegetables in a diet is very helpful in burning body fat.

Avocado Toast with Crushed Peanuts

This simple food item contains a lot of healthy fat and fiber. All you need to do is toast a slice of bread and spread the avocado onto it. You can add spices for your taste too.

Chicken, Vegetable or Bean Soup

Soups allow you to take in a maximum amount of nutrition. All the goodness of the ingredients that you add gets added up in the soup.

Avocado/Chicken/Vegetable Salad

Preparation method

Raw vegetables have more nutrition than roasted or fried ones. You can add dressings and spices of your choice to make a delicious salad. Including chicken, meat and avocado in your salad will increase the nutritional profile of your lunch.

Chickpea Salad

Chickpeas make a great replacement for meat in a vegetarian or vegan diet. They reduce the risk of several diseases, improve digestion and help in weight loss.

Tuna Pita Sandwiches

Tuna has amazing benefits for your body. Your tuna sandwich will be healthy if you do not dress it up with mayonnaise and baked bread.

Broccoli Slaw Salad

Boiled broccoli prevents many diseases. A person wanting to lose weight must have broccoli on his/her shopping list.

Dinner

The final meal of the day should be light yet fulfilling. It should boost metabolism and increase the digestion since you will not be eating until the next day. Meals that you can use for your meal plan are given below.

Spicy Chicken Chili

Spices, chicken, and chili peppers are all good for your body. They help in losing weight and increasing muscles and metabolism. They form a very enriching and fulfilling dinner.

Quinoa Salad

Quinoa is one of the healthiest and most nutritious foods that exist. It is rich in fibers, protein and amino acids, which are great for weight loss.

Shrimp Fried Rice

This low-fat food contains fibers and proteins. It makes a very healthy yet tasty choice for dinner. Vegetarians and vegans can add broccoli and soybeans instead of shrimp to their fried rice.

Lemon Garlic Chicken Drumsticks

Lemon, garlic, and chicken boost your metabolism and clear the stored waste inside the body.

Seafood

Fish, salmon, anchovies, tuna, and char are all rich in omega-3 fatty acids. They are great for your heart, brain, and bones.

Roasted Vegetables

They can be a part of your lunch and dinner alike, based on your mood, IF plan and taste.

Steak

Steak is loaded with protein and is good for your waistline. Make sure you get lean cuts of this red meat to keep the calorie intake low.

Snack Time

There are times between the big meals when your stomach craves food. Satisfy your hunger by eating food that is light and low in calories. Go for these healthy snacks when you crave food between your meals. Each of them is high in nutritional value and will help you to feel full for a longer time.

- Fruit of Choice (Apple, Banana, Berries)

- Almonds

- Protein Bar

- Yogurt

- Edamame

- Carrots

- Zucchini Chips

- Cottage Cheese

- Low-Sugar Ice Cream

- Lemon juice

Meal Plan

There are seven days in a week, and you have already been provided with more than seven options for each of your meals. You can now make your meal planaccording to your liking and taste. Choose the meals that you would prefer, design your 7-day plan, and stick to it to achieve maximum weight loss.

FAQS

Now that you have basic knowledge related to intermittent fasting, you may still feel overwhelmed and intimidated. You might have a range of questions in mind and want to confirm if you should proceed.

Undoubtedly, losing weight is not an easy task. It needs dedication and firm belief in the diet plan that you are following. Most diet plans focus most on the different types of food that one must consume.

This is where intermittent fasting is unique. Intermittent fasting is a method which instead of regulating the amount and type of food that one is consuming, regulates the time of consumption. However, as we have already discussed, intermittent fasting does not affect women and men in the same way.

In this section, we will answer your common queries in detail.

How is intermittent fasting done?

When one opts for intermittent fasting, usual eating times are punctuated by short-term fasts. This ensures that not too many unnecessary calories are consumed. But intermittent fasting does not primarily involve monitoring how many calories are being consumed regularly or what the macronutrient intake is each day.

This method is more of a system that should be incorporated into one's lifestyle than adiet.

Intermittent fasting can be done in many ways, and one can choose whichever seems most convenient. The three most common ways of intermittent fasting are:

- Fasting on every alternate day

- Fasting for sixteen hours every day, and then breaking the fast with a wholesome meal

- Fasting for a whole day

- Fasting only twice a week

Now, even though intermittent fasting can be done in many ways, women should consult a doctor before choosing a method, especially if they have any nutritional deficiencies, fertility problems, irregular periods, have had certain eating disorders in the past, are expecting or are breastfeeding. In all these cases, the doctor might suggest some specific changes in the methods or introduce a different diet for the days during which one is not fasting.

What are the best ways of intermittent fasting for women?

A modified approach to intermittent fasting is advisable for women because there can be certain side effects if one is not cautious. The following are the methods which are best for women.

- Crescendo Method: This method requires one tofast for about 12 to 16 hours, twice or thrice a week. But the cycle should be maintained, and the days of fasting should be after proper intervals that cannot be disrupted.

- Leangains Method (16/8 method): Usually, in this method, one must fast for about 16 hours and then consume a specific number of calories within 8 hours. However, for women, it is advisable that initially a 14-hour fast is held before increasing it gradually to 16 hours.

- Modified Alternate Day Fasting: A much more relaxed method, this way of intermittent fasting allows one to fast only on certain days of the week while following a completely normal diet on the other days, without any restrictions on the calorie intake. Also, on a fasting day, when the fast is broken, 20-25% of the usual number of calories can be consumed.

- The 24-hour Protocol: Also known as the Eat-Stop-Eat method, this requires one to fast for a whole day, twice a week (women should not attempt this more than two times a week). The best way to approach this method is to start fasting for about 16 hours and then slowly increase the time.

- The Fast Diet: This method requires one to keep track of the daily calorie intake. On fasting days (twice a week), the calorie intake should be restricted to 20-25% of the usual intake, while on other days, one can eat normally. Since the fast is done on two days, while a normal diet is followed during the other five, this way of intermittent fasting is also known as the 5:2 method.

All these methods are beneficial for women, and they have minimal side effects. If followed properly, they will not cause any issues. Here, it is important to keep in mind that no matter which method one chooses to follow, a proper diet should be maintained on the non-fasting days, otherwise it can take a toll on one's health.

However, if too many oily, fatty foods are consumed on the non-fasting days, then it will be difficult to observe any significant change in body weight or the overall lifestyle, even after a long period of time.

How does intermittent fasting affect women? What are its benefits and side effects?

While it is overall a very effective method, intermittent fasting has caused problems, especially in women (as mentioned before) and it has not been very beneficial to some. Given below are certain points that explain the problems in detail.

According to several studies, intermittent fasting has caused significant disruption in the blood sugar levels. This has been observed only in women and not in men. For many women, blood sugar levels have been seen to be out of control, and the situations have only worsened as they continue with their fasting.

Intermittent fasting can affect the menstrual cycle. Many women have complained that once they started intermittent fasting, their menstrual cycles became irregular, and some even experienced cramps and pain.

The reason for this maybe the body's sensitivity towards calorie restriction, which is common in women. If very few calories are consumed, then the secretion of the gonadotropin-releasing hormone (GnRH) is affected. The gonadotropin-releasing hormone triggers the release of two other hormones: luteinizing hormone (LH) and the follicle-stimulating hormone (FSH). Now, any disruption in the release of these hormones will directly affect the menstrual cycle and cause irregular periods, deterioration of bone health, and even infertility.

The points mentioned above are two of the major problems that some women face when they follow a strict routine of intermittent fasting. To avoid such side effects, it is advisable that women take a different approach towards intermittent fasting, which will include very short fasts to maintain proper calorie intake. Also, women should avoid fasting for a whole day.

Now, while there are side effects, intermittent fasting does help women a lot with their lifestyle patterns. There are many health benefits of intermittent fasting in women, and not all of them involve losing weight. These benefits have been discussed below.

Heart diseases are usually caused by high LDL cholesterol levels, or high blood pressure or high triglyceride levels. Recent studies have shown that intermittent fasting in women (especially overweight women) can reduce high blood pressure by 6% in around eight weeks. Intermittent fasting can also reduce LDL cholesterol levels by almost 25% and triglyceride levels by 35%, which immediately results in reducing the risk of heart disease.

An increase in insulin levels, in turn, increases insulin resistance in one's body, which can cause diabetes. For women, intermittent fasting can reduce insulin levels and insulin resistance. It has been seen in recent studies that if intermittent fasting is done over a certain period of time (about twelve weeks), then insulin levels will be lowered by almost 30%.

Now, as mentioned before, intermittent fasting for women is not very effective in the case of blood sugar levels and does cause disruption. But it can still reduce high blood sugar levels in women by about 5%, and this is beneficial to those who have pre-diabetes (a condition where blood sugar levels are high but not as high as they would be in a diabetic patient).

Intermittent fasting is usually done to lose weight. If one fasts for a short period of time, then it is easier not to consume too many calories. This way, one will not end up eating any more than what is necessary. For women, intermittent fasting is an effective way to lose weight; and sometimes it works better than the diets that restrict calorie intake.

For obese females, a study has shown that intermittent fasting for about 3 months led to a weight loss of up to 7 kg. Another study has shown that when intermittent fasting is done for a shorter period (for about a few weeks), then it is observed that the bodyweight is reduced by 3-8%.

Apart from the aforementioned benefits, intermittent fasting also helps in reducing chronic inflammation, binge eating disorders (which, in turn, lowers depression and creates a better lifestyle), and it also helps in retention of muscle mass, which results in the burning of more calories, even while resting.

Intermittent fasting is a simple and easy way to combat obesity. For women, it is necessary to follow a relaxed version of intermittent fasting and then gradually build up to longer hours of fasting. This way, it becomes quite safe and convenient. The method of intermittent fasting is not complicated, but it needs to be followed without any sudden changes to yield proper health benefits.

RECIPES

Breakfast recipes

Choco Chip Whey Waffles

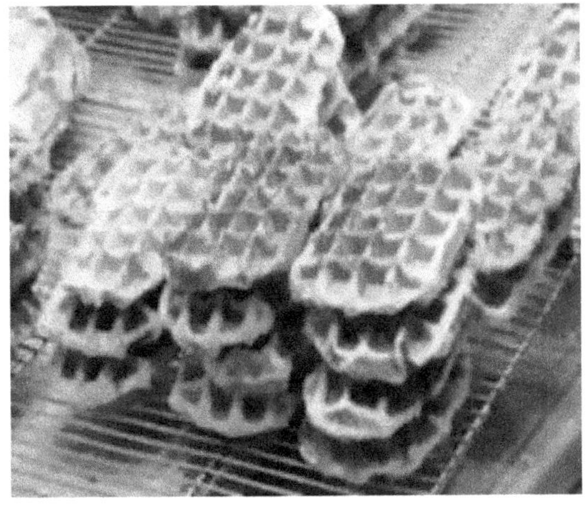

Serves:2

Prep time: 10 minutes

Cooking Time: 6 minutes

Ingredients:

- 2-tbsp organic coconut oil

- 2-tbsp coconut sugar

- 4-tbsp chocolate whey protein powder

- ⅓-cup almond flour

- A pinch of salt

- ½-tsp baking powder

- ½-cup almond milk

- 2-pcs eggs

Directions:

1. Mix all the ingredients in the blender to obtain a homogenous paste.

2. Preheat your waffle iron. Pour the waffle dough in the iron and cook each waffle for 3 minutes.

Nutritional Values per Serving:

Calories: 423

Fat: 32.8g

Protein: 26.5g

Total Carbohydrates: 8.3g

Dietary Fiber: 2.9g

Net Carbohydrates: 5.4g

Coco Cinnamon-Packed Pancakes

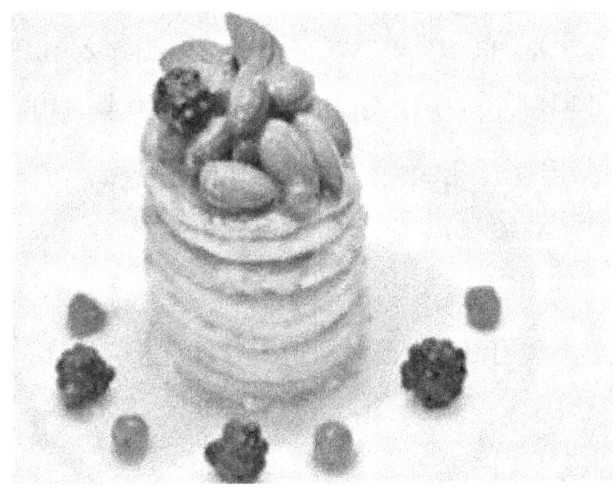

Serves:2

Prep time: 30 minutes

Cooking Time: 5 minutes

Ingredients:

- 2-pcs eggs

- 2½-tbsp organic coconut flour

- ¼-cup milk substitute with hydrogenated vegetable oil (or almond milk)

- 1-tbsp baking soda

- ½-tbsp cinnamon

- ½-tbsp baobab powder

- 2-tbsp organic coconut flower syrup

Directions:

1. In a salad bowl, mix the coconut flour, baobab powder, cinnamon, and baking soda.

2. Add the beaten eggs, the almond milk, and the coconut syrup. Let the dough rest for 30 minutes.

3. Cook the pancakes in a hot pan with coconut oil.

4. Dress the pancakes with raspberries/blueberries or almonds.

Nutritional Values per Serving:

Calories: 392

Fat: 32.5g

Protein: 20g

Total Carbohydrates: 11.3g

Dietary Fiber: 6.4g

Net Carbohydrates: 4.9g

Magdalena Muffins with Tart Tomatoes

Serves:2

Prep time: 10 minutes

Cooking Time: 20 minutes

Ingredients:

- 2½-tbsp whole-wheat flour

- 2½-tbsp almond flour

- 1-tbsp yeast or baking soda

- A dash of salt, pepper, and paprika

- 2-pcs eggs

- 1-tbsp organic cashew nuts

- 1-tbsp hemp oil

- 2½-tbsp soymilk

- ⅓-cup feta cheese, diced

- 1⅓-cup dried tomatoes, without oil and sliced into small pieces

Directions:

1. Mix the wheat flour, almond flour, yeast, and spices.

2. Then add eggs, cashews, oil, and soymilk.

3. Mix well to obtain a smooth paste. Add the feta and tomatoes.

4. Mix well and pour the dough into muffin pans previously greased with coconut oil.

5. Bake for 20 minutes at 350°F.

Nutritional Values per Serving:

Calories: 405

Fat: 33.3g

Protein: 20.3g

Total Carbohydrates: 11g

Dietary Fiber: 4.9g

Net Carbohydrates: 6.1g

Spinach Shoots Mediterranean Medley

Serves: 2

Prep time: 10 minutes

Cooking Time: 1 minute

Ingredients:

- ½-cup spinach shoots
- 2-tbsp quinoa
- ¼-cup avocado, sliced
- 1-tbsp fresh goat cheese
- 1-tsp agave syrup, gluten-free
- ¼-cup dried blackberries
- 1-pc fig
- 1-tsp pumpkin seeds puree

Directions:

1. Arrange the spinach shoots, cooked quinoa, and avocado on a large plate.

2. Mix the goat cheese, agave syrup, and dried blackberries.

3. Make 4 small cuts in the fig so that you can open it and insert the goat cheese mixture.

4. Spread your fig on the spinach shoots. Sprinkle over with pumpkin seed puree.

Nutritional Values per Serving:

Calories: 308

Fat: 26g

Protein: 15.4g

Total Carbohydrates: 9.7g

Dietary Fiber: 6.5g

Net Carbohydrates: 3.2g

Romantic Raspberry Power Pancake

Serves:1

Prep time: 5 minutes

Cooking Time: 10 minutes

Ingredients:

- 2-tbsp raspberries, crushed

- 2-tsp almond flour

- 1-tbsp yeast or baking soda

- 1-tbsp vegan protein powder

- 2-tbsp soymilk

- 1-tbsp coconut oil

Directions:

1. Mix the crushed raspberries and dry ingredients.

2. Pour the milk and mix well to obtain a homogenous mixture.

3. Cook the pancakes for 2 minutes on each side using a little coconut oil in a pan. Flip the pancake when small bubbles appear.

4. Dress with almonds or nuts.

Nutritional Values per Serving:

Calories: 323

Fat: 25.3g

Protein: 15.7g

Total Carbohydrates: 12g

Dietary Fiber: 3.8g

Net Carbohydrates: 4.8g

Spinach Sausage Feta Frittata

Serves: 6

Prep Time: 15 minutes

Cooking Time: 30 minutes

Ingredients:

- 10-oz. spinach, frozen, thawed, drained, and chopped

- 12-oz. sausage, sliced into small pieces

- ½-cup feta cheese, crumbled

- ½-cup almond milk, unsweetened

- ½-cup heavy cream

- ¼-tsp. ground nutmeg

- ½-tsp. salt

- ¼-tsp. black pepper

- 12-pcs eggs, whisked

Directions:

1. Place the sausage in a medium-sized mixing bowl. Break the spinach up into the same bowl as the sausage.

2. Sprinkle the cheese over the mixture. Toss lightly until fully combined. Lightly spread

the mixture onto a greased 13" × 9" casserole dish, or greased muffin cups.

3. In a larger bowl, blend the almond milk, cream, nutmeg, salt, and pepper with the eggs, and mix well until fully combined.

4. Gently pour the mixture into the dish or muffin cups until for about ¾ full. Bake at 375°F for about 50 minutes (for the casserole), or 30 minutes (for the muffin cups), or until fully set.

Nutritional Values per Serving:

Calories: 295

Fat: 22.9g

Protein: 18.5g

Total Carbohydrates: 4.6g

Dietary Fiber: 1g

Net Carbohydrates: 3.6g

Mayonnaise Mixed with Energy Egg

Serves: 1

Prep Time: 2 minutes

Cooking Time: 5 minutes

Ingredients:

- 2-tbsp organic mayonnaise, gluten-free

- 1-pc large egg

- 1-tbsp butter

Directions:

1. Mix the mayonnaise and egg in a medium-sized bowl until fully combined.

2. Melt the butter in a non-stick skillet. Pour the egg mixture, and cook until set. Scrape the egg and all remaining fat onto a serving plate. Serve immediately.

Nutritional Values per Serving:

Calories: 295

Fat: 22.7g

Protein: 18.8g

Total Carbohydrates: 3.8g

Dietary Fiber: 0.1g

Net Carbohydrates: 3.7g

Avocados atop Toasted Tartiné

Serves: 2

Prep Time: 10 minutes

Cooking Time: 5 minutes

Ingredients:

- 2-slices bread, gluten-free
- ½-pc small avocado, thinly sliced
- 1-tbsp fresh cheese
- 1-tsp lemon juice
- A dash of salt and pepper
- 1-tsp chia seeds for garnish (optional)

Directions:

1. Toast lightly the bread slices.

2. Carefully arrange the avocado slices on each bread slice. Drizzle with the lemon juice. Spread the fresh cheese. Sprinkle with pepper and salt. Top with garnish.

Nutritional Values per Serving:

Calories: 268

Fat: 22.4g

Protein: 13.5g

Total Carbohydrates: 8.9g

Dietary Fiber: 6.7g

Net Carbohydrates: 3.2g

Fish Fillet & Perky Potato Cheese Combo

Serves: 2

Prep Time: 15 minutes

Cooking Time: 10 minutes

Ingredients:

- 1-tbsp olive oil

- 1-pc large potato, cooked and thinly sliced

- ¼-cup lean white cheese

- ½-tsp herbs of your choice

- 3.5-oz. herring fillet, steamed and sliced in half

- ½-tsp flaxseed oil or coconut oil

- A dash of salt and pepper

Directions:

1. Heat a non-stick pan with olive oil. Add potato slices and cook for several minutes until browned.

2. Season the white cheese with salt, pepper, and herbs of your choice.

3. Arrange the potatoes equally between two plates. Top with the cheese and herring fillets. Garnish with a drizzle of flaxseed oil.

Nutritional Values per Serving:

Calories: 298

Fat: 24.9g

Protein: 14.2g

Total Carbohydrates: 6.5g

Dietary Fiber: 3.2g

Net Carbohydrates: 4.3g

Cream Cheese Protein Pancake

Serves: 2

PrepTime: 10 minutes

Cooking Time: 12 minutes

Ingredients:

- 2-pcs eggs

- 2-oz cream cheese

- 1-packet sweetener

- ½-tsp cinnamon

- 1-tbsp butter

Directions:

1. Mix all the ingredients in a blender except the butter. Blend until smooth. Let the batter stand for 2 minutes to allow the bubbles to settle.

2. Grease slightly a hot pan with ¼-tbsp butter. Pour ¼-batter into the pan. Cook for about 2 minutes until turning golden. Flip the pancake and cook for 1 minute on its other side.

3. Repeat the same cooking procedure with the remaining batter. Serve with fresh berries of choice and sugar-free syrup.

Nutritional Values per Serving:

Calories: 340

Fat: 28.1g

Protein: 16.2g

Total Carbohydrates: 8.1g

Dietary Fiber: 3.8g

Net Carbohydrates: 4.3g

Veggie Variety with Peanut Paste

Serves: 1

Prep Time: 15 minutes

Cooking Time: 15 minutes

Ingredients:

- 1-bulb small onion, thinly sliced
- ¾-cup broccoli, sliced into quarters
- 1-pc small carrot, sliced into quarters
- ½-pc green pepper, thinly sliced
- 5-pcs mushrooms, sliced into quarters
- A dash of salt, pepper, and powdered chili
- 2-tbsp peanut butter, dairy-free
- 2-tbsp. soy sauce, gluten-free
- 1-tbsp agave syrup (or honey), gluten-free
- ¼-cup red cabbage, thinly sliced

Directions:

1. Pour a little water in a heated skillet and cook the onions until they are transparent. Add the broccoli, carrot, pepper, and mushrooms. Cook for 10 minutes until tender. (Add some water if the pan is too dry). Season the veggies with a dash of salt, pepper, and chili.

2. For the sauce, mix the peanut butter with the soy sauce, agave syrup, and 3 tbsp water.

3. To serve, incorporate the red cabbage. Garnish the dish with the sauce.

Nutritional Values per Serving:

Calories: 349

Fat: 28.7g

Protein: 18.4g

Total Carbohydrates: 10.8g

Dietary Fiber: 6.5g

Net Carbohydrates: 4.3g

Avocado Aliment with Egg Element

Serves: 2

Prep Time: 8 minutes

Cooking Time: 20 minutes

Ingredients:

- 1 egg, whisked

- 1 avocado, halved, pitted, and removed slightly with flesh

- A dash of sea salt and pepper

- 1-tbsp parsley, chopped

- 1-tsp cayenne pepper

Directions:

1. Preheat your oven to 375°F.

2. Pour the egg gently into each halved avocado. Remove the excess liquid.

3. Place the stuffed avocado in a baking tray. Bake for 20 minutes.

4. Season the preparation with sea salt, parsley, and cayenne pepper.

Nutritional Values per Serving:

Calories: 275

Fat: 23.8g

Protein: 11.8g

Total Carbohydrates: 10.7g

Dietary Fiber: 4g

Net Carbohydrates: 3.4g

Pumpkin Pancakes

Serves: 3

Prep Time: 10 minutes

Cooking Time: 30 minutes

Ingredients:

- 1-tsp vanilla extract

- 1-cup coconut cream

- 3-pcs eggs

- 2-tbsp egg whites

- ½-cup pumpkin puree

- 5-packs sweetener

- 4-tbsp ground flax seed

- 4-tbsp ground hazelnuts or hazelnut flour

- 1-tsp yeast or baking powder

- 1-tbsp black tea powder

- 1-tbsp. coconut oil for cooking

Directions:

1. Whisk together the first five liquid ingredients for half a minute until they become frothy. Mix the dry ingredients in a separate bowl.

2. Combine both the dry and liquid ingredients to obtain a batter. (Add water, as necessary if the mixture is too thick.)

3. Grease a saucepan with a teaspoon of coconut oil. Ladle in the first pancake.

4. Cover the pan and cook for 3 minutes. Flip and cook the other side.

5. Repeat the cooking process until using up all the batter.

Nutritional Values per Serving:

Calories: 200

Fat: 16.4g

Protein: 11g

Total Carbohydrates: 5.2g

Dietary Fiber: 3g

Net Carbohydrates: 2.2g

Whole-Wheat Plain Pancakes

Serves: 1

Prep Time: 5 minutes

Cooking Time: 12 minutes

Ingredients:

- 2-pcs eggs

- 4-tbsp whole-wheat flour

- ½-tsp yeast or baking soda

- ⅓-cup sunflower oil

- 1-tbsp coconut oil for cooking

Directions:

1. Mix all the ingredients in a bowl until obtaining a smooth consistency.

2. Pour the coconut oil in a pan placed over medium heat. Cook for 3 minutes until browned. Flip and cook the other side.

3. Serve hot and garnish with fresh fruits of your choice such as blueberries, strawberries or raspberries, nuts, and coconut flakes.

Nutritional Values per Serving:

Calories: 329

Fat: 27.6g

Protein: 16.1g

Total Carbohydrates: 5.4g

Dietary Fiber: 1.3g

Net Carbohydrates: 4.4g

Blueberries Breakfast Bowl

Serves: 1

Prep Time: 35 minutes

Cooking Time: 0 minutes

Ingredients:

- 1-tsp chia seeds

- 1-cup almond milk

- ¼-cup fresh blueberries or fresh fruits

- 1-pack sweetener for taste

Directions:

1. Mix the chia seeds with almond milk. Stir periodically.

2. Place in the fridge to cool for 30 minutes, and then serve with fresh fruit. Enjoy!

Nutritional Values per Serving:

Calories: 202

Fat: 16.8g

Protein: 10.2g

Total Carbohydrates: 9.8g

Dietary Fiber: 5.8g

Net Carbohydrates: 2.6g

Feta-Filled Tomato-Topped Oldie Omelet

Serves: 1

Prep Time: 5 minutes

Cooking Time: 6 minutes

Ingredients:

- 1-tbsp coconut oil
- 2-pcs eggs
- 1½-tbsp milk
- A dash of salt and pepper
- ¼-cup tomatoes, sliced into cubes
- 2-tbsp feta cheese, crumbled

Directions:

1. Beat the eggs with the pepper, salt, milk, and the remaining spices.

2. Pour the mixture into a heated pan with coconut oil.

3. Stir in the tomatoes and cheese. Cook for 6 minutes or until the cheese melts.

Nutritional Values per Serving:

Calories: 335

Fat: 28.4g

Protein: 16.2g

Total Carbohydrates: 4.5g

Dietary Fiber: 0.8g

Net Carbohydrates: 3.7g

Ave Avocado Super Smoothie

Serves: 1

Prep Time: 10 minutes

Cooking Time: 1 minute

Ingredients:

- ½-cup Greek yogurt
- 7-oz. frozen avocados
- ½-cup water
- ½-tsp vanilla powder
- 1-tsp each chia seeds, chocolate chips, and peanut butter for garnish

Directions:

1. Mix all the ingredients. You can also use a blender to crush them.

2. Pour the smoothie into a bowl and garnish to your taste with fruits, seeds or nuts.

Nutritional Values per Serving:

Calories: 398

Fat: 33.1g

Protein: 20g

Total Carbohydrates: 15.5g

Dietary Fiber: 10.6g

Net Carbohydrates: 4.9g

Hearty Hodgepodge

Serves: 1

PrepTime: 5 minutes

Cooking Time: 25 minutes

Ingredients:

- 1-bulb small onion, diced

- 1-tbsp coconut oil

- 1-tbsp bacon bits

- 1-pc medium zucchini, diced into squares

- 1-tbsp parsley or chives, chopped

- ¼-tsp. of salt

- 1-pc large egg, fried

Directions:

1. Sauté the onion with coconut oil in a pan placed over medium heat. Add the bacon, stirring frequently until both onion and bacon turn slightly brown.

2. Add the zucchini, and cook for 15 minutes. Remove from heat and transfer the preparation in a serving bowl. Sprinkle over the parsley.

3. To serve, top the dish with the fried egg.

Nutritional Values per Serving:

Calories: 290

Fat: 24g

Protein: 14.6g

Total Carbohydrates: 6.7g

Dietary Fiber: 3.1g

Net Carbohydrates: 3.6g

Chocolate Chia Plain Pudding

Serves: 3

Prep Time: 55 minutes

Cooking Time: 0 minutes

Ingredients:

- 3-tbsp chia seeds

- 2-cups water

- ¼-cup whey chocolate protein

- ½-cup Greek yogurt, sugar-free

- ¼-cup linseeds, roasted

- 1-tbsp cocoa powder, unsweetened

- 1-packet sweetener (optional)

Directions:

1. Add chia seeds to a bowl of water and let stand for 20 minutes whileoccasionally stirring.

2. When chia seeds are inflated, add the other ingredients and mix again.

3. Refrigerate for 30 minutes before serving.

Nutritional Values per Serving:

Calories: 370

Fat: 28.7g

Protein: 22.3g

Total Carbohydrates: 10.8g

Dietary Fiber: 5.2g

Net Carbohydrates: 5.6g

Seasoned Sardines with Sunny Side

Serves: 1

PrepTime: 5 minutes

Cooking Time: 10 minutes

Ingredients:

- 2-oz. sardines in olive oil

- 2-pcs eggs

- ½-cup arugula

- ¼-cup artichoke hearts, diced

- A pinch of salt

- A dash of black pepper

Directions:

1. Preheat your oven to 375°F.

2. Place the sardines in an oven-ready stoneware bowl. Add the eggs on top of the sardines. Top the eggs with the arugula and artichokes. Sprinkle with salt and pepper.

3. Bake for 10 minutes until the eggs cook through.

Nutritional Values per Serving:

Calories: 255

Fat: 21g

Protein: 13.5g

Total Carbohydrates: 4.9g

Dietary Fiber: 1.8g

Net Carbohydrates: 3.1g

Healthy Breakfast Burritos

Serves: 4

Prep time - 5 mins

Cooking time - 10 mins

Ingredients

- 8 eggs

- 1 tbsp milk

- 1 tbsp garlic, minced

- 1 red pepper, minced

- Half an onion, red if possible, minced

- 4 slices of bacon, cooked

- Salt

- Pepper

- 4 tortilla wraps (multi-grain or wholegrain)

- little cheese (optional)

Directions:

1. Take a medium-sized saucepan and heat over a medium heat

2. Add the garlic and cook for a couple of minutes, until fragrant

3. Whisk the eggs with the milk and place to one side

4. Add the pepper and onion to the pan and allow to cook for a couple more minutes

5. Add the eggs to the pan and cook for 4 minutes

6. Once cooked, add a quarter of the egg mixture onto each tortilla wrap and add one piece of the bacon on top

7. You can add cheese if you want, although it isn't necessary

8. Wrap up and enjoy it!

Nutritional Values per Serving:

Calories: 352

Carbs: 22g

Fat: 20g

Protein: 8g

LUNCH RECIPES

Pulled Pepper-Lemon Loins

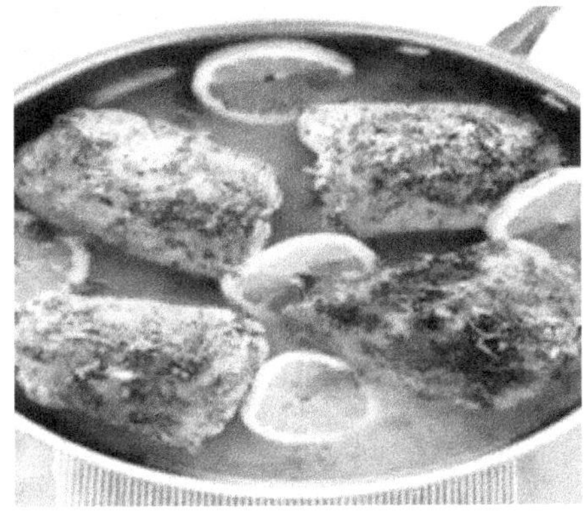

Serves: 4-servings

Prep time: 15 minutes

Cooking Time: 240-360 minutes

Ingredients

- ½-stick of butter

- 1-pc large lemon, sliced

- 1-pc green pepper, chopped

- 1-tbsp garlic, minced

- 2-tbsp olive oil

- 1-tbsp salt

- 1-tsp dried thyme

- ½-tbsp Dijon mustard
- 3-lbs. (4-pcs) chicken tenderloins
- 1-cheddar cheese slice, shredded
- 4-leaves romaine lettuce

Directions:

1. Combine the butter, lemon, pepper, garlic, oil, salt, thyme, and mustard in your slow cooker. Switch the slow cooker on high and melt the butter.

2. Add the chicken; ensure to coat the chicken with the butter mixture.

3. Cook on high for 4 hours or on low for 6 hours. Add the cheese and let it sit for 15 minutes on low.

4. To serve, place the chicken over a bed of lettuce leaves.

Nutritional Values per Serving:

Calories: 280

Fat: 23.3g

Protein: 14g

Total Carbohydrates: 4.1g

Dietary Fiber: 0.6g

Net Carbohydrates: 3.5g

Shrimps & Spinach Spaghetti

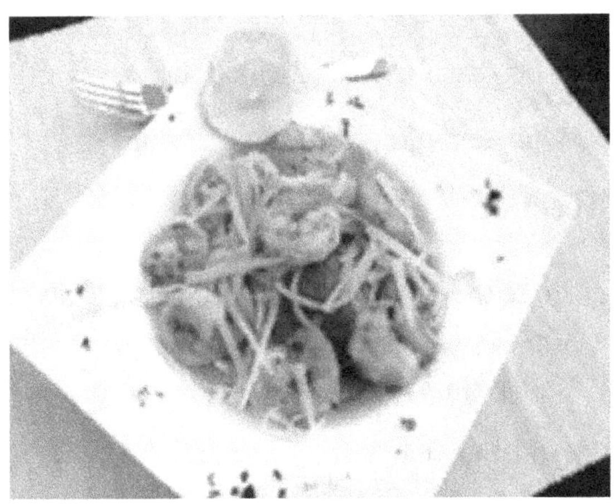

Serves: 2

Prep time: 5 minutes

Cooking Time: 8 minutes

Ingredients:

- 8-tbsp vegetable broth

- 1-cup low carb spaghetti, rinsed and drained

- 1-pc leek, cut into strips

- 1⅓-cup frozen peas

- 1⅓-cup fresh spinach leaves

- ¼-lb. shrimp, pre-cooked

- 1-tbsp lemon zest

- 1-pc green pepper, finely chopped (divided, per serving)

- 2-pcs basil leaves (divided, per serving)

- 1-pc lemon (divided, per serving)

Directions:

1. Pour the vegetable broth in a wok and cook for 5 minutes. Add the leeks, peas, spinach, and shrimp. Cook further for 5 minutes.

2. Add the spaghetti, and continue cooking for 2 minutes. Remove quickly from heat and pour into a bowl, mix with lemon zest.

3. Divide the pasta equally between two plates. To serve, garnish with the pepper, basil leaves, and lemon.

Nutritional Values per Serving:

Calories: 425

Fat: 33g

Protein: 25g

Total Carbohydrates: 15.7g

Dietary Fiber: 10.4g

Net Carbohydrates: 5.3g

Single Skillet Seafood-Filled Frittata

Serves:4

Prep time: 2 minutes

Cooking Time: 18 minutes

Ingredients:

- 1-pc green pepper

- ¼-pc lime, squeezed for juice

- 1-tbsp coconut flour

- 1-tbsp sesame oil

- 1-tbsp soy sauce, gluten-free

- 1-tbsp coconut oil

- 3-bulbs fresh onions, chopped

- ½-clove garlic, minced

- ¼-cup prawns, raw

- 1⅓-cup mussels, deshelled

- 2-pcs eggs, whisked

Directions:

1. Preheat your oven to 475°F. Meanwhile, make the sauce by combining the first five ingredients in a mixing bowl. Mix thoroughly until fully combined. Set aside.

2. Melt the coconut oil in a small skillet and fry the onions. Add the garlic, prawns, and mussels. Cook for 10 minutes until the prawns turn pink.

3. Stir in the eggs. Place the skillet in the oven and bake for 5 minutes.

4. Slice the frittata in four slices and serve with the sauce.

Nutritional Values per Serving:

Calories: 459

Fat: 38.2g

Protein: 22.9g

Total Carbohydrates: 8.7g

Dietary Fiber: 3g

Net Carbohydrates: 5.7g

Poultry Pâté & Creamy Crackers

Serves:1

Prep time: 15 minutes

Cooking Time: 35 minutes

Ingredients:

- 3.5-oz. chicken livers

- 3-tbsp butter, softened

- 1-tsp. Italian seasoning

- A pinch of salt and pepper

- 3-pcs unsalted creamy crackers, gluten-free

Directions:

1. Put all the ingredients in a blender apart from the crackers. Blend to a smooth paste consistency.

2. Serve with the crackers.

Nutritional Values per Serving:

Calories: 437

Fat: 36.4g

Protein: 21.9g

Total Carbohydrates: 5.5g

Dietary Fiber: 0g

Net Carbohydrates: 5.5g

Chickpeas Carrots Curry

Serves:1

Prep time: 5 minutes

Cooking Time: 25 minutes

Ingredients:

- ½-bulb onion, finely chopped

- ½-pc carrot, sliced into cubes

- ½-tsp coconut oil

- ¼-cup chickpeas

- ½-tsp tomato paste

- 3-tbsp light soy cream

- ½-tsp turmeric powder

- ⅛-bunch fresh coriander

- A pinch of salt, pepper, and sweet paprika

Directions:

1. Sauté the onions and carrots for 5 minutes with coconut oil in a skillet.

2. Add the chickpeas, tomato paste, soy cream, turmeric, coriander, and spices. Mix well and cook for 10 minutes.

3. Cook the rice for 10 minutes in boiling water. Serve the konjac rice with the vegetable curry and chickpeas.

Nutritional Values per Serving:

Calories: 380

Fat: 30.9g

Protein: 18g

Total Carbohydrates: 14.4g

Dietary Fiber: 10.7g

Net Carbohydrates: 3.7g

Baked Broccoli in Olive Oil

Serves: 3

Prep Time: 5 minutes

Cooking Time: 25 minutes

Ingredients:

- 1½-lbs broccoli florets

- ¼-cup olive oil

- 3-tsps. garlic, minced

- 2-tbsp fresh basil, chopped

- ½-tsp red chili flakes

- ¾-tsp kosher salt

- Zest of ½-pc lemon

- Juice of ½-pc lemon

- ⅓-cup parmesan cheese

Directions:

1. Preheat your oven to 425°F.

2. Arrange the broccoli florets in a baking sheet lined with parchment paper.

3. Season the broccoli with olive oil, chopped fresh basil, minced garlic, kosher salt, red chili flakes, zest and juice of half a lemon each.

4. Sprinkle parmesan cheese over the broccoli. Place the sheet in the oven to bake for about 25 minutes.

Nutritional Values per Serving:

Calories: 484

Fat: 39.2g

Protein: 26.7g

Total Carbohydrates: 21.6g

Dietary Fiber: 16.8g

Net Carbohydrates: 4.8g

Bunless Bacon Burger

Serves: 4

Prep Time: 8 minutes

Cooking Time: 37 minutes

Ingredients:

- 1½-lbs. ground beef
- 2-tbsp olive oil
- 2-tbsp bacon bits
- 4-oz. pepper jack cheese
- 1-bulb onion, sliced crosswise
- 8-leaves romaine lettuce
- A dash of salt and pepper

Directions:

1. Form the ground beef into four patties. Cook for 4 minutes with olive oil on a skillet placed over medium heat. Flip the patties to cook the other sides. Set aside.

2. Using the same skillet, stir-fry the bacon bits for 5 minutes until crispy.

3. Use the lettuce leaves as buns. Place each patty on a leaf and top with the bacon bits. Sprinkle a dash of salt and pepper. Top each burger with the cheese to melt.

Nutritional Values per Serving:

Calories: 435

Fat: 36.3g

Protein: 21.7g

Total Carbohydrates: 6.1g

Dietary Fiber: 0.7g

Net Carbohydrates: 5.4g

Smoky Sage Sausage

Serves: 4

Prep Time: 5 minutes

Cooking Time: 8 minutes

Ingredients:

- 2-tbsp sage, chopped
- 2-packets sweetener
- 1-tsp salt
- 1-tsp maple extract
- 1-lb. ground pork
- ½-tsp black pepper
- ¼-tsp garlic powder
- ⅛-tsp cayenne pepper

Directions:

1. Mix all the ingredients in a mixing bowl.
2. Form patties from the mixture.
3. Put the patties in a skillet placed over medium heat. Cook for 4 minutes until cooked through. Flip the patties to cook on the other side.

Nutritional Values per Serving:

Calories: 170

Fat: 13.2g

Protein: 8.4g

Total Carbohydrates: 5.3g

Dietary Fiber: 1g

Net Carbohydrates: 4.3g

Steamed Salmon & Salad Bento Box

Serves: 2

Prep Time: 10 minutes

Cooking Time: 0 minutes

Ingredients:

- 2-pcs salad heads

- 1-cup carrot, grated

- ¼-cup cucumber, sliced

- 1-pc green pepper, thinly sliced

- 4-cups marinara pasta, rinsed, drained, and cooked for 2 minutes in boiling water

- ½-lb. salmon, steamed

- 2-pcs lemons

- 2-pcs eggs, boiled and sliced

- 1-tsp chia seeds

- 4-tbsp yogurt, sugar-free

- 1-tsp turmeric powder

- ½-pc lemon, zest

- 2-tbsp mint, minced

- A pinch of pepper

Directions:

1. Divide equally the first eight ingredients between two bento boxes. Sprinkle the arrangements with chia seeds.

2. Mix the rest of the ingredients to make the sauce. Pack the sauce separately.

Nutritional Values per Serving:

Calories: 391

Fat: 30.4g

Protein: 24.9g

Total Carbohydrates: 11.8g

Dietary Fiber: 7.3g

Net Carbohydrates: 4.5g

Stuffed Spaghetti Squash

Serves: 2

Prep Time: 30 minutes

Cooking Time: 30 minutes

Ingredients:

- 1-pc spaghetti squash, halved and pitted

- 1-tsp olive oil

- ½-cup bacon strips, grilled

- 3-cups ground beef

- 1-pc green pepper, thinly sliced

- ½-bulb onion, sliced into cubes

- 1-tsp garlic powder

- 1-tsp paprika

- A pinch of salt and pepper

- 1-cup cheddar cheese, grated

Directions:

1. Rub the squash halves with oil, and bake for 30 minutes at 350°F.

2. Meanwhile, roast the bacon in a saucepan placed over high heat. Stir in the onion and pepper. Add the beef and spices. Use salt and

pepper to season the mixture and cook for 15 minutes, stirring regularly. Set aside.

3. Remove the flesh of the cooked squash by scratching with a fork. Mix the flesh with the meat mixture. Add the cheese, and put the mixture in the frayed squash.

4. Return the stuffed squash to the hot oven, and bake for 10 minutes.

Nutritional Values per Serving:

Calories: 404

Fat: 33.2g

Protein: 20.3g

Total Carbohydrates: 7g

Dietary Fiber: 1g

Net Carbohydrates: 6g

Prawn Pasta

Serves: 3

PrepTime: 10 minutes

Cooking Time: 12 minutes

Ingredients:

- 1-tsp sesame seeds

- 1-pc lime

- ½-pc green pepper, thinly sliced

- 2 tbsp coconut flour

- 2-tbsp sesame oil

- 1-tbsp soy sauce, gluten-free

- 2-heads small cabbages

- 6-bulbs small onions, chopped

- 1-cup prawns, steamed

- 3-cups low-carb pasta, rinsed, drained, and cooked for 2 minutes in boiling water

- 8-pcs small radishes, sliced into 4-pieces for garnish

- ½-pc avocado, sliced for garnish

Directions:

1. Mix the first six ingredients in a bowl to make the pasta sauce. Set aside.

2. Cook the cabbage for 10 minutes in a pan with a little water and soy sauce. Add the onions and prawns. Cook for 2 minutes.

3. Arrange the pasta in a plate, topped with the prawn mixture, pasta sauce, and the garnishing.

Nutritional Values per Serving:

Calories: 393

Fat: 32.8g

Protein: 19.7g

Total Carbohydrates: 14.9g

Dietary Fiber: 10.1g

Net Carbohydrates: 4.8g

Tasty Tofu Carrots &Cauliflower Cereal

Serves: 1

Prep Time: 20 minutes

Cooking Time: 20 minutes

Ingredients:

For the Tofu-Carrots Mix:

- ½-block extra firm tofu, crumbled

- 2-tbsp reduced sodium soy sauce, gluten-free

- ½-cup onion, diced

- 1-cup carrot, diced

- 1-tsp turmeric

For the Cauliflower Cereal:

- 3-cups riced cauliflower

- 2-tbsp reduced sodium soy sauce, gluten-free

- 1½-tsp toasted sesame oil

- 1-tbsp rice vinegar

- 1-tbsp ginger, minced

- ½-cup broccoli, finely chopped

- 2-cloves garlic, minced

- ½-cup frozen peas

Directions:

1. Toss the tofu with the rest of the tofu-carrots mix ingredients. Place the mixture in your air fryer basket. Lock the lid and cook for 10 minutes at 370°F.

2. Meanwhile, toss together all of the cauliflower cereal ingredients. Add this mixture to the air fryer pan. Lock the lidand cook for another 10 minutes at 375°F.

Nutritional Values per Serving:

Calories: 390

Fat: 32.6g

Protein: 19.5g

Total Carbohydrates: 17.4g

Dietary Fiber: 12.7g

Net Carbohydrates: 4.7g

Stuffed Straw Mushroom Mobcap

Serves: 1

Prep Time: 15 minutes

Cooking Time: 5 minutes

Ingredients:

- 1-cup fresh spinach, washed, bathed in ice, and drained

- 1-cup straw mushrooms or Chinese mushroom, washed and stems removed

- 1-tbsp coconut oil

- 1-bulb onion, finely chopped

- 1-clove garlic, minced

- A dash of salt and pepper

- A pinch of nutmeg

- ¼-cup quinoa, cooked

- 3.5-oz. cottage cheese

Directions:

1. Spread the spinach leaves over the food film while rolling them.

2. Fry the mushrooms with coconut oil in a saucepan before adding onion and garlic.

Season with pepper, salt and nutmeg. Set aside.

3. Combine the cooked quinoa with the cottage cheese. Spread the mixture evenly on the spinach leaves then roll into a pudding with the help of the food film.

4. Stuff the mushroom heads with the spinach pudding, and place them in the fridge.

5. Just before serving, slice the mushroom head with a sharp knife and pass quickly to the pan to heat.

Nutritional Values per Serving:

Calories: 401

Fat: 34.7g

Protein: 17.2g

Total Carbohydrates: 16.9g

Dietary Fiber: 11.4g

Net Carbohydrates: 5g

Crispy Chicken Packed in Pandan

Serves: 4

PrepTime: 30 minutes

Cooking Time: 18 minutes

Ingredients:

- 4-pcs (½-lb.) chicken thigh
- 1-tbsp shallot
- 1-pc lemon
- 1-tsp of fennel seeds
- 1-tsp of turmeric powder
- 1-tsp of chili powder
- 1-tbsp of oyster sauce, gluten-free
- A pinch of salt
- A pinch of sugar
- A handful of pandan leaves

Directions:

1. Preheat your air fryer to 350°F for about 5 minutes.

2. Marinate the chicken with all the ingredients. Set aside for 30 minutes.

3. Wrap each chicken meat with the pandan leaves.

4. Arrange the wrapped chicken in the air fryer basket and lock the lid

5. Set to cook for 18 minutes at 375°F.

Nutritional Values per Serving:

Calories: 382

Fat: 32.5g

Protein: 17.8g

Total Carbohydrates: 7.7g

Dietary Fiber: 3.1g

Net Carbohydrates: 4.6g

Chicken Curry Masala Mix

Serves: 3

Prep Time: 10 minutes

Cooking Time: 35 minutes

Ingredients:

- 2-tbsp sesame oil (divided)

- 2-tbsp ginger, diced

- 1½-lbs chicken thighs, boneless, skinless, and diced

- 1-cup tomatoes, chopped

- ¼-cup coriander, chopped

- 2-tsp turmeric

- 1-tsp cumin

- 1-tsp cayenne

- 2-tbsp lemon juice

- Cilantro or mint leaves for garnish

Directions;

1. Sauté the ginger and jalapeno pepper with half of the sesame oil in a saucepan. Add the. Stir in the chicken, tomatoes, and coriander. Add the spices, the remaining sesame oil, lemon juice and half a cup of water.

2. Cover and cook for 30 minutes.

3. To serve, pour everything in a deep salad bowl, and garnish with cilantro or mint leaves.

Nutritional Values per Serving:

Calories: 377

Fat: 29.3g

Protein: 23.4g

Total Carbohydrates: 6.8g

Dietary Fiber: 1.9g

Net Carbohydrates: 4.9g

Milano Meatballs with Tangy Tomato

Serves: 3

Prep Time: 25 minutes

Cooking Time: 30 minutes

Ingredients:

For the Meatballs:

- 1-lb extra-lean ground beef

- 1-pc egg, whisked

- 10-pcs sun-dried tomatoes, chopped

- ½-cup ricotta cheese

- 1-cup Parmigiano-Reggiano cheese or parmesan cheese, freshly grated

- salt and freshly ground black pepper

For the Tomato Sauce:

- 1-bulb onion, finely chopped

- ¼-cup extra-virgin olive oil

- 2-lbs. tomato puree, gluten-free

- A pinch of salt and freshly ground black pepper

Directions:

1. Combine all the meatball ingredients in a mixing bowl. Mix well until fully combined. Form balls from the mixture, and pat them down for even cooking.

2. Sauté the onions with olive oil in a skillet until they are translucent. Add the tomato puree and bring to a boil. Add the remaining ingredients and the meatballs. Cook for 30 minutes on medium heat.

Nutritional Values per Serving:

Calories: 396

Fat: 32.6g

Protein: 20.9g

Total Carbohydrates: 8.2g

Dietary Fiber: 3.4g

Net Carbohydrates: 4.8g

Aubergine À la Lasagna Lunch

Serves: 2

Prep Time: 20 minutes

Cooking Time: 30 minutes

Ingredients:

- 2-pcs large eggplants, sliced and drained from excess liquid with a paper towel

- A pinch of sea salt

- 2-cups part-skim ricotta cheese

- ½-cup parmesan cheese, freshly grated

- 1-pc egg, whisked

- 4-cups homemade tomato sauce, sugar-free

- 2-tbsp part-skim mozzarella cheese, shredded

- 2-tbsp cheddar cheese, grated

- 2-tbsp parsley, chopped

Directions:

1. Preheat your oven to 375°F. Meanwhile, season the eggplant slices with salt. Grill the eggplant slices for 3 minutes on each side.

2. Combine the ricotta, parmesan, and egg in a large bowl. Set aside.

3. Spread half of the tomato sauce in a saucepan. Layer half of the eggplant slices, and top with half of the cheddar and mozzarella. Pour half of the ricotta mixture over the layer, or just enough to coat it.

4. Cover the saucepan and insert it into your preheated oven. Bake for 25 minutes. Set to cool for 10 minutes.

5. Repeat the process for the second lasagna set. To serve, garnish your lasagna with chopped parsley

Nutritional Values per Serving:

Calories: 346

Fat: 27g

Protein: 21.4g

Total Carbohydrates: 7.9g

Dietary Fiber: 3.5g

Net Carbohydrates: 4.4g

Beef Broccoli with Sesame Sauce

Serves: 4

Prep Time: 10 minutes

Cooking Time: 45 minutes

Ingredients:

- 2-tbsp coconut oil

- 1-tsp arrowroot powder

- 1-tbsp sesame oil

- 1-tbsp redfish sauce

- ½-tsp light sea salt

- ¼-tsp black pepper

- ¼-tsp baking powder

- 1-lb. beef, sliced into ¼-inch thick chunks

- 2-tsp sesame oil or olive oil

- 1-head broccoli, diced

- 2-tbsp coconut oil

- 2-cloves garlic, minced

- 2-ginger, finely chopped

- A pinch of salt and pepper

Directions:

1. Mix the first seven ingredients in a bowl to make the sesame sauce. Set aside.

2. Fry the meat with sesame oil for 15 minutes until browned.

3. In a saucepan with water, add the broccoli, oil, garlic, and ginger. Season it with a pinch of salt and pepper. Add and spread the fried beef with the broccoli. Cover and cook for 20 minutes. Pour the sauce and cook for 10 more minutes.

Nutritional Values per Serving:

Calories: 375

Fat: 31g

Protein: 19.5g

Total Carbohydrates: 5.4g

Dietary Fiber: 0.8g

Net Carbohydrates: 4.6g

Sautéed Sirloin Steak in Sour Sauce

Serves: 4

Prep Time: 10 minutes

Cooking Time: 30 minutes

Ingredients:

- 1-bulb medium onion, chopped

- 1-clove garlic, minced

- 2-tbsp butter

- 1-lb. sirloin steak, trimmed and cut into thin strips

- ½-tsp salt

- ¼-tsp pepper

- 1-tbsp thyme

- 1½ cup fresh mushrooms, sliced

- 1-tbsp red wine vinegar

- 1-(10.5 oz.) can cream of mushroom soup

- 2-tbsp sour cream

- 4-cups egg noodles, cooked according to package instructions

Directions:

1. Sauté the onion and garlic with melted butter in a large skillet placed over medium heat. Remove from pan and set aside.

2. Add the beef strips, salt, pepper, and thyme. Cook evenly over low heat until browned.

3. Return the onion and garlic, and stir in the mushrooms, wine vinegar, and soup. Cover and simmer for 7 minutes until mushrooms are tender. Uncover and add sour cream. Stir and heat through. Serve immediately over the prepared noodles.

Nutritional Values per Serving:

Calories: 350

Fat: 29.3g

Protein: 17.7g

Total Carbohydrates: 4.9g

Dietary Fiber: 1g

Net Carbohydrates: 3.9g

Flaky Fillets with Garden Greens

Serves: 4

Prep Time: 25 minutes

Cooking Time: 30 minutes

Ingredients:

- 1-lb broccoli, chopped into cubes and seasoned with a dash of salt and pepper

- 2-tbsp coconut oil

- 7-pcs scallions

- 2-tbsp small capers

- 1-tbsp sesame oil or olive oil

- 1½-lbs. white fish, sliced into 4 fillets

- 1-tbsp dried parsley

- 1¼-cups whipping cream, gluten-free and sugar-free

- 1-tbsp mustard, sugar-free

- 1-tsp of salt

- ¼-tsp ground black pepper

- ⅓-cup olive oil

- 5-oz. leafy greens

Directions:

1. Sauté the seasoned broccoli with sesame oil in a pan, and add the scallions and capers. Add the fish in the middle of the sautéed greens. Simmer for 15 minutes.

2. Meanwhile, mix the parsley with the whipping cream and mustard. Pour it over the cooked fish and vegetables. Drizzle with a little bit of coconut oil.

3. Return the saucepan on medium heat and cook for an extra 10 minutes.

Nutritional Values per Serving:

Calories: 395

Fat: 33g

Protein: 19.8g

Total Carbohydrates: 8.7g

Dietary Fiber: 3.9g

Net Carbohydrates: 4.8g

DINNER RECIPES

Pizza Pie with Cheesy Cauliflower Crust

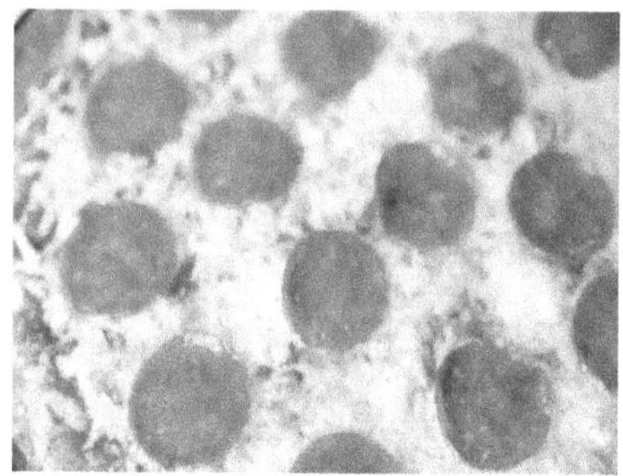

Serves:2

Prep time: 5 minutes

Cooking Time: 30 minutes

Ingredients:

- ½-head cauliflower, rinsed, riced, cooked for 5 minutes in boiling water, and drained

- 2-pcs eggs, whisked

- ⅓-parmesan cheese

- ½-cup cherry tomatoes, washed and halved

- 2-tbsp organic hempseed oil

- 1-tsp balsamic vinegar

- 1-mozzarella cheese ball, crumbled

- ¼-cup basil leaves

Directions:

1. Spin the cooked cauliflower in a dishtowel to let out as much liquid as possible. (The goal is to obtain a flour texture.) Add the eggs and cheese. Mix well.

2. Spread to a disk the cauliflower dough on a baking pan lined with parchment paper. Bake for 15 minutes at 400°F in your preheated oven.

3. Meanwhile, mix the tomatoes with hempseed oil and balsamic vinegar. Season the mixture with salt and pepper.

4. Remove the pizza dough from the oven. Add the tomato mixture and sprinkle over with mozzarella. Return the pan in the oven and bake further for 15 minutes.

5. Serve hot and garnish with fresh basil leaves.

Nutritional Values per Serving:

Calories: 384

Fat: 32.1g

Protein: 19.9g

Total Carbohydrates: 5.5g

Dietary Fiber: 1.7g

Net Carbohydrates: 3.8g

Roasted Rib-eye Skillet Steak

Serves: 2

Prep time: 5 minutes

Cooking Time: 15 minutes

Ingredients:

- 1-16oz rib-eye steak (1 to 1¼-inch thick)

- 2-tbsp duck fat or peanut oil (divided)

- A dash of salt and pepper

- 1-tbsp butter

- ½-tsp thyme, chopped

Directions:

1. Preheat your oven to 400°F. Place a cast iron skillet inside.

2. Season the rib-eye steak with oil, salt, and pepper.

3. Take the preheated skillet out from the oven and place over the stove, set in medium heat. Pour oil, and add the steak. Sear for 2 minutes on both sides.

4. Return the skillet with the steak in the oven. Roast for 6 minutes.

5. Remove the skillet and place over the stove, set in low heat. Add the butter and thyme in

the skillet. Baste the steak for about 4 minutes.

Nutritional Values per Serving:

Calories: 722

Fat: 60.2g

Protein: 45g

Total Carbohydrates: 0g

Dietary Fiber: 0g

Net Carbohydrates: 0g

À la Spaghetti with Asian Sauce

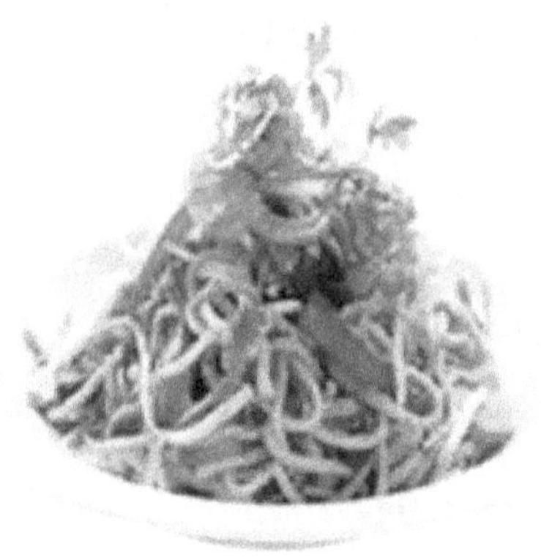

Serves: 2

Prep time: 10 minutes

Cooking Time: 15 minutes

Ingredients:

For the Sauce:

- 2-tbsp soy sauce, gluten-free

- 1-tsp of hemp oil

- 1-tsp of lemon juice

- 1-tbsp peanut butter

For the Spaghetti:

- ½-bulb onion, diced

- 1-tsp coconut oil

- 1-tsp red or green pepper, diced

- 1-pc carrot, thinly sliced lengthwise

- 1 egg, whisked

- 5-oz. low-carb spaghetti, rinsed and cooked for 2 minutes in boiling water

- Fresh coriander and peanuts for garnish

Directions:

1. Combine all the sauce ingredients in a bowl. Set aside.

2. Sauté the onion with oil, and add the peppers, carrots, egg, sauce, and spaghetti. Cook for 13 minutes, stirring frequently.

3. To serve, garnish with fresh coriander and peanuts.

Nutritional Values per Serving:

Calories: 412

Fat: 34.4g

Protein: 20.9g

Total Carbohydrates: 10.5g

Dietary Fiber: 5.7g

Net Carbohydrates: 4.8g

Shirataki& Soy Sprouts Pad Thai with Peanut Tidbits

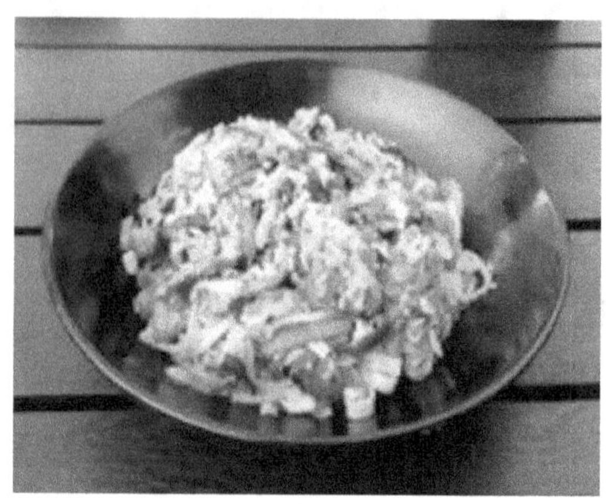

Serves:1

Prep time: 10 minutes

Cooking Time: 5 minutes

Ingredients:

For the Sauce:

- 1-tbsp peanut butter

- 2-tbsp soy sauce, gluten-free

- ½-lime

- 2-tbsp agave syrup, gluten-free

- ½-tbsp organic turmeric

For the Noodles:

- 1-bag of konjacshirataki noodles, rinsed and cooked for 2 minutes in boiling water

- 1-pc carrot, thinly sliced

- 1-bulb onion, thinly sliced

- ½-cup soy sprouts

- ¼-cup unsalted peanuts

- Some sprigs of fresh coriander

Directions:

1. Combine all the sauce ingredients in a bowl. Set aside.

2. Heat the pasta with a little coconut oil in a frying pan. Pour the sauce and add the coriander. Mix well and cook for 5 minutes.

3. To serve, place in a bowl and garnish with peanuts and coriander sprigs.

Nutritional Values per Serving:

Calories: 423

Fat: 35.2g

Protein: 21g

Total Carbohydrates: 14.9g

Dietary Fiber: 9.6g

Net Carbohydrates: 5.3g

Charred Chicken with Squash Seed Sauce

Serves:1

Prep time: 15 minutes

Cooking Time: 20 minutes

Ingredients:

For the Sauce:

- 2-tbsp white almond puree

- 2-cloves of garlic, finely chopped (divided, for the sauce and chicken marinade)

- ½-tbsp squash seeds

- 1-tbsp barley

- 1-pc fresh basil

For the Marinade:

- 2-branches rosemary, finely chopped

- 1-pc red chili, finely chopped

- 1-pc lemon (keep the zest)

- Pinch of salt and ground black pepper

- 1-tbsp olive oil

- 1-cup chicken breasts, cubed

- 5-bulbs small onions, sliced in quarters

- 5-pcs cherry tomatoes

Directions:

1. Combine and mix all the sauce ingredients in a bowl. Set aside.

2. Mix all the marinade ingredients and let stand for 10 minutes. Thread alternately the onions, meat, and tomatoes into the skewers and grill over a coal fire for 10 minutes on each side. Serve the chicken kebabs with the squash seed sauce.

Nutritional Values per Serving:

Calories: 428

Fat: 35.6g

Protein: 21g

Total Carbohydrates: 16.9g

Dietary Fiber: 11.6g

Net Carbohydrates: 5.3g

Therapeutic Turmeric &Shirataki Soup

Serves: 1

Preparation Time: 10 minutes

Cooking Time: 32 minutes

Ingredients:

- 1-tbsp turmeric powder
- 1-serving chicken-vegetable broth soup
- 3-pcs carrots, sliced into small pieces
- 3-slices ginger
- 1-pack (5-oz.) konjacshirataki noodles
- ¼-lb. chicken breast, sliced into strips

Directions:

1. Simmer all the ingredients over low heat for 30 minutes.

2. Rinse the konjac noodles thoroughly under cold water.

3. Add the noodles to the broth and heat for 2 minutes.

Nutritional Values per Serving:

Calories: 415

Fat: 34.6g

Protein: 21.6g

Total Carbohydrates: 10.1g

Dietary Fiber: 5.7g

Net Carbohydrates: 4.4g

Fresh Fettuccine with Pumpkin Pesto

Serves: 3

Prep Time: 15 minutes

Cooking Time: 2 minutes

Ingredients:

For the Pesto Sauce:

- 1-tbsp olive oil

- 1-tbsp pumpkin seed oil

- ½-tsp pumpkin seeds

- ¼-cup barley

- 1-tbsp lemon juice

- A pinch salt

For the Pasta:

- 1¾-cup zucchini, washed, peeled, and cut into thin noodle strips

- ½-cup cherry tomatoes, washed and cut in half

- 1¼-cup low carb fettuccine

- 1-pc mozzarella cheeseball

- A pinch of pepper

Directions:

1. Combine and mix all the sauce ingredients with 2-tbsp water in a bowl. Set aside.

2. Boil the fettuccine for 1 minute and add the zucchini. Boil further for another minute, and drain.

3. Toss the pasta with the pesto sauce. Season the dish with a pinch of pepper and garnish with tomatoes and mozzarella.

Nutritional Values per Serving:

Calories: 417

Fat: 34.7g

Protein: 20.9g

Total Carbohydrates: 10.5g

Dietary Fiber: 5.3g

Net Carbohydrates: 5.2g

Cheddar Chicken Casserole

Serves: 6

Prep Time: 10 minutes

Cooking Time: 30 minutes

Ingredients:

* 20-oz. chicken breasts

* 2-tbsp olive oil (divided)

* 2-cups broccoli, steamed

* ½-cup sour cream

* ½-cup heavy cream

* 1-oz. pork rinds, crushed

* A dash of salt and pepper

* ½-tsp paprika

* 1-tsp oregano

* 1-cup cheddar cheese, grated

Directions:

1. Preheat your oven to 450°F.

2. Sear the chicken with a tablespoon of olive oil in a pan until it cooks all the way through. Shred the meat in the pan. Add the remaining oil, broccoli, and sour cream.

3. Place and spread evenly the mixture in an 8"
    x11" pan. Press firmly and drizzle with
    heavy cream. Add all the remaining
    seasonings and top the casserole with the
    cheese. Place the pan in the oven and bake
    for 25 minutes until the edges turn brown and
    start bubbling.

Nutritional Values per Serving:

Calories: 405

Fat: 33.8g

Protein: 22.7g

Total Carbohydrates: 3.6g

Dietary Fiber: 1g

Net Carbohydrates: 2.6g

Zesty Zucchini Pseudo Pasta & Sweet Spanish Onions Overload

Serves: 2

Prep Time: 10 minutes

Cooking Time: 20 minutes

Ingredients:

- 2-tbsp of vegetable oil

- 2-pcs yellow onions or Spanish onions

- 1-tbsp low-sodium soy sauce

- 2-tbsp low-sodium teriyaki sauce

- 1-tbsp sesame seeds

- 4-pcs small zucchinis, sliced into spaghetti strips using a spiral cutter

Directions:

1. Add the vegetable oil, onions, and soy sauce to a saucepan placed over medium heat. Stir in the teriyaki sauce and sesame seeds. Mix well until fully combined.

2. Cook for 10 minutes, stirring frequently until the vegetables turn brown.

3. Add the zucchini pasta and cook for 3 minutes.

4. To serve, transfer the pasta in a serving dish and garnish with chopped parsley.

Nutritional Values per Serving:

Calories: 319

Fat: 25.9g

Protein: 18.1g

Total Carbohydrates: 6.6g

Dietary Fiber: 3.2g

Net Carbohydrates: 3.4g

Soba & Spinach Sprouts

Serves: 2

Prep Time: 15 minutes

Cooking Time: 0 minutes

Ingredients:

- 3-pcs mushrooms, sliced into quarters

- ⅓-cup smoked tofu, sliced into squares

- 1-tbsp coconut oil

- ½-pc green pepper, sliced into strips

- 3-tbsp cashew nuts

- ½- clove garlic

- ½-pc lime, juice

- A dash of salt and pepper

- ¼-cup water (more, as needed)

- ¼-cup soba noodles, cooked according to package instructions

- 1⅓-cup spinach sprouts

- 1-tbsp coconut shavings for garnish

Directions:

1. Fry the mushrooms and tofu with coconut oil in a frying pan until they turn brown. Add the pepper. Set aside.

2. For the sauce, mix cashews with garlic, lime juice, salt, pepper, and a little water.

3. Divide the noodles between two bowls and top with spinach sprouts. Arrange the remaining vegetables on top. Garnish with coconut shavings or avocado slices, sesame seeds, and a slice of lime.

4. To serve, pour over the sauce on each arranged bowl.

Nutritional Values per Serving:

Calories: 355

Fat: 29.6g

Protein: 17.8g

Total Carbohydrates: 8.3g

Dietary Fiber: 3.9g

Net Carbohydrates: 4.4g

Chickpeas & Carrot Consommé

Serves: 2

Prep Time: 10 minutes

Cooking Time: 20 minutes

Ingredients:

- ¼-lb. chickpeas, cooked

- 1-tbsp coconut oil

- 1-clove garlic, minced

- 1-piece ginger, minced

- 1-bulb small onion, finely chopped

- ½-lb. carrots, sliced into small pieces

- 1¼-cup vegetable broth

- A dash of salt and pepper

- ½-cup coconut milk

- 1-tbsp coconut shaving

Directions:

1. Arrange the chickpeas on a plate lined with parchment paper. Sprinkle with salt, curry, and paprika. Spread the spices well and bake for 15 minutes at 350°F.

2. Melt the coconut oil in a saucepan and brown the garlic, ginger, and onion. Add the carrots.

Deglaze with vegetable broth and simmer for 15 minutes over medium heat until the carrots cook through.

3. Season to taste with salt, pepper, curry, and paprika. Pour the coconut milk.

4. Mix the soup and garnish with chickpeas and coconut shavings.

Nutritional Values per Serving:

Calories: 460

Fat: 38.2g

Protein: 23.3g

Total Carbohydrates: 10.1g

Dietary Fiber: 4.3g

Net Carbohydrates: 5.8g

Chicken Cauliflower Curry

Serves: 2

PrepTime: 15 minutes

Cooking Time: 30 minutes

Ingredients

- 1-cup vegetable broth
- 1-tbsp curry paste
- ½-cup light coconut milk
- ½-lb chicken breast, cooked and sliced into small pieces
- 1-pc potato, diced
- 1-clove garlic, minced
- ½-bulb onion, finely chopped
- 1-cup cauliflower, diced
- ⅓-cup fresh peas
- Salt and pepper
- ¼-cup goji berries

Directions:

1. Heat the vegetable broth in a wok for 5 minutes. Add the curry paste, coconut milk, meat, potato, garlic, and onion. Cook for 15 minutes.

2. Add the vegetables and cook further for 10 minutes until they are tender. Season the curry with a dash of salt and pepper.

3. To serve, garnish with goji berries.

Nutritional Values per Serving:

Calories: 334

Fat: 27g

Protein: 18.7g

Total Carbohydrates: 8.4g

Dietary Fiber: 4.3g

Net Carbohydrates: 4.1g

Cheesy Cauliflower Mac Munchies

Serves: 2

Prep Time: 20 minutes

Cooking Time: 15 minutes

Ingredients:

- 1-pc medium cauliflower, riced

- 3-tbsp + ½-tsp avocado oil (divided)

- A pinch of sea salt

- A pinch of black pepper

- 1-cup cheddar cheese, shredded

- ¼-cup cream, gluten-free

- ¼-cup almond milk, unsweetened

Directions:

1. Preheat your air fryer to 400°F. Spray the pan with oil.

2. Place the riced cauliflower in the pan and drizzle with the avocado oil. Toss well and season with a pinch each of salt and pepper. Set aside.

3. Heat the cheese, cream, and milk with a little bit of avocado oil in a pot.

4. Pour the cheese mixture over the seasoned cauliflower. Lock the lid of the air fryer and set to cook for 14 minutes.

Nutritional Values per Serving:

Calories: 352

Fat: 27.8g

Protein: 20.9g

Total Carbohydrates: 8.9g

Dietary Fiber: 4.3g

Net Carbohydrates: 4.6g

Sugar Snap Pea Pods with Coco Crunch

Serves: 2

Prep Time: 5 minutes

Cooking Time: 10 minutes

Ingredients:

- 4-tbsp salted butter, gluten-free and dairy-free

- 1-tbsp coconut oil

- ½-cup coconut, unsweetened and shredded

- ⅛-tsp cinnamon

- 1-tbsp rosemary oil

- 9-oz. snap pea pods, trimmed, strings removed, and diced

- A pinch of salt

Directions:

1. In a saucepan, melt the coconut oil with the butter over medium heat. Add the coconut shreds, rosemary oil, and cinnamon. Toss very well until fully incorporated.

2. Add the diced pea pods and mix again. Leave to cook for 8 minutes until the pea pods start to melt.

3. To serve, sprinkle over a pinch of salt.

Nutritional Values per Serving:

Calories: 389

Fat: 31.3g

Protein: 22g

Total Carbohydrates: 7.2g

Dietary Fiber: 2.3g

Net Carbohydrates: 4.9g

Spicy & Smoky Spinach-Set Fish Fillets

Serves: 2

Prep Time: 15 minutes

Cooking Time: 10 minutes

Ingredients:

- 2-pcs halibut meat (11-oz. each), membrane removed and deboned

- 4-cups packed spinach

- Juice of ½-pc lemon

- A pinch of salt and pepper

- A pinch of smoked paprika

- 1-pc sliced lemon

- 1-pc green onions, sliced

- 1-pc red chili, deseeded and thinly sliced

- 1-cup cherry tomatoes, halved

- 2-tbsp avocado oil

Directions:

1. Place the halibut meat over a flat surface. Divide the spinach between them.

2. Lay each halibut meat on each pile of spinach. Squeeze the lemon over each part and season with smoked paprika.

3. Top each fish meat with lemon slices, green onions, chili, and the cherry tomatoes. Pour 1-tbsp of avocado oil over each fish portion.

4. Wrap around each fish meat tightly with foil; arrange them in a baking pan. Cook for 10 mins until the fish turns golden and flaky when forked.

Nutritional Values per Serving:

Calories: 248

Fat: 18.8g

Protein: 15.3g

Total Carbohydrates: 13.2g

Dietary Fiber: 8.9g

Net Carbohydrates: 4.3g

Spicy Shrimps & Sweet Shishito

Serves: 2

Prep Time: 15 minutes

Cooking Time: 15 minutes

Ingredients:

- 2-tbsp canola oil

- A pinch of sea salt

- 1-clove garlic, crushed and finely chopped

- 1-pc red chili pepper, seeded and finely chopped

- 5-oz. whole shishito peppers

- 10-oz. shrimps, jumbo size

- 1-tsp sesame oil

- 2-tbsp low-sodium light soy sauce

- Juice of 1-pc lime

Directions:

1. Preheat your air fryer to 350°F for about 5 minutes. Spray your air fryer pan with canola oil.

2. Add the salt, garlic, and red chili pepper. Mix well until fully combined.

3. Add the shishito peppers; mix thoroughly again. Add the shrimps and drizzle with sesame oil.

4. Place the pan in your air fryer and lock the lid. Cook for about 10 minutes at 400°F

5. Divide the dish equally between three serving bowls. To serve, season each bowl with lime juice and soy sauce.

Nutritional Values per Serving:

Calories: 370

Fat: 28.9g

Protein: 23g

Total Carbohydrates: 7.2g

Dietary Fiber: 2.8g

Net Carbohydrates: 4.4g

SPAGHETTI-STYLED ZESTY ZUCCHINI WITH GUACAMOLE GARNISH

Serves: 2

Prep Time: 15 minutes

Cooking Time: 5 minutes

Ingredients:

- 2-pcs medium zucchini, cut into spaghetti strips using a spiral cutter

- 1-tbsp sea salt

- 1-pc large avocado, peeled, pitted, and cut into small pieces

- 1⅓-cup fresh basil, washed, dried and finely chopped

- 2-tbsp lemon juice

- A dash of salt and black pepper

- 1-tbsp coconut oil

- 7-oz. mushrooms, cleaned and cut into slices

- 1-pc pomegranate, seeds extracted

Directions:

1. Season the zucchini strips with sea salt and set aside.

2. Mix the avocado slices, lemon juice, and a dash of salt and pepper. Set aside.

3. Toss lightly the zucchini in a frying pan placed over medium heat. Fry for 4 to 5 minutes in coconut oil. Add the mushrooms and pomegranate seeds.

4. To serve, place the zucchini spaghetti on a plate with the avocado cream in a separate bowl. Garnish with the basil leaves.

Nutritional Values per Serving:

Calories: 381

Fat: 31.8g

Protein: 19g

Total Carbohydrates: 14.3g

Dietary Fiber: 9.5g

Net Carbohydrates: 4.8g

Grain-less Gnocchi in Melted Mozzarella

Serves: 1

Prep Time: 10 minutes

Cooking Time: 15 minutes

Ingredients:

- 2-cups mozzarella, shredded

- ½-tsp garlic powder

- 1-tsp salt

- 3-pcs large egg yolks, whisked (divided)

- ½-cup tomato sauce, gluten-free

Directions:

1. Melt the mozzarella with the garlic powder and salt for 5 minutes in a microwave-safe dish.

2. Pour half of the egg yolks into the mozzarella mixture in a large bowl. Mix until fully combined. Add the remaining egg yolks. Mix thoroughly again until fully incorporated.

3. Divide the mixture into four parts. Roll each part into a long rope over a flat surface. Cut each rope into gnocchi-like pieces, pressing each with a fork.

4. Bring a pan filled with water to a boil. Add the gnocchi dumplings and cook for about 2 minutes.

5. Preheat your air fryer to 350°F. Spray the air fryer pan with cooking oil.

6. Arrange the gnocchi pieces in the air fryer pan. Lock the lid of the air fryer and cook for 10 minutes.

7. To serve, pour the tomato sauce over the gnocchi.

Nutritional Values per Serving:

Calories: 355

Fat: 27.6g

Protein: 22.1g

Total Carbohydrates: 6.5g

Dietary Fiber: 2.1g

Net Carbohydrates: 4.4g

Cauliflower Chao Fan Fried with Pork Pastiche

Serves: 4

Prep Time: 20 minutes

Cooking Time: 15 minutes

Ingredients:

- ½-head medium-sized cauliflower, chopped into small cubes
- 2-pcs eggs
- 2-cloves garlic, chopped
- 2-cups pork belly, cut into thin strips
- 3-pcs green capsicums
- 2-bulbs onions
- 1-tbsp soy sauce, gluten-free
- 1-tsp black sesame seeds
- 1-tbsp spring onion, chopped
- 1-tsp pickled ginger

Directions:

1. Place the chopped cauliflower in your food processor; pulse into smaller granules. Set aside.

2. Whisk the eggs, and swirl in the frying pan. Cook for 3 minutes.

3. Add the pork belly strips and the cauliflower rice. Stir in the onions and soy sauce. Cook for about 10 minutes.

4. To serve, distribute the preparation equally between four serving bowls. Garnish with sesame seeds, spring onions, and pickled ginger.

Nutritional Values per Serving:

Calories: 460

Fat: 35.7g

Protein: 28.6g

Total Carbohydrates: 8.3g

Dietary Fiber: 2.3g

Net Carbohydrates: 6g

All-Avocado Stuffed with Spicy Beef Bits

Serves: 6

Prep Time: 20 minutes

Cooking Time: 20 minutes

Ingredients:

- 1-lb. ground beef
- 1-tbsp chili powder
- ½-tsp salt
- ¾-tsp cumin
- ½-tsp dried oregano
- ¼-tsp garlic powder
- ¼-tsp onion powder
- 4-oz. tomato sauce, gluten-free
- 3-pcs medium-sized avocados, halved and pitted
- 1-cup cheddar cheese, shredded for garnish
- ¼-cup cherry tomatoes, sliced for garnish
- ¼-cup lettuce, shredded for garnish
- A dash of chopped cilantro for garnish

Directions:

1. Cook the beef with oil and a little water in a pan for 10 minutes, stirring frequently until it

turns brown. Stir in the spices and tomato sauce. Cook for another 10 minutes.

2. Load the cooked beef to each halved avocado and top with garnish.

Nutritional Values per Serving:

Calories: 280

Fat: 23.1g

Protein: 14g

Total Carbohydrates: 6.3g

Dietary Fiber: 2.2g

Net Carbohydrates: 4.1g

SNACKS

Coconut Candy

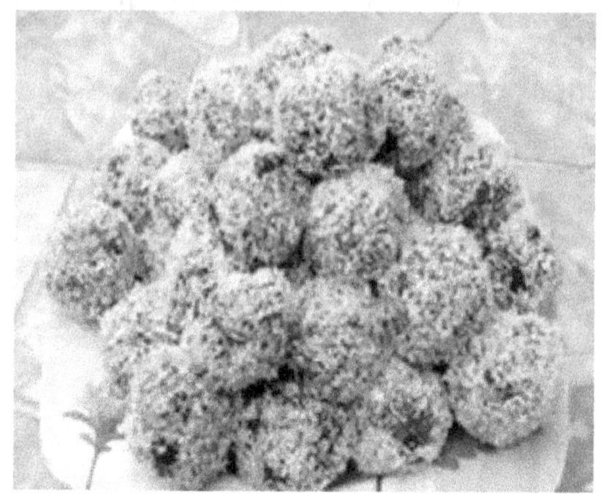

Serves: 1

Prep time: 10 minutes

Cooking Time: 0 minutes

Ingredients:

- 2-tbsp coconut butter (or notably known as Coconut Manna)

Directions:

1. Melt the coconut butter at room temperature until it resembles a creamy butter consistency.

2. Spoon out the melted butter into candy molds. Refrigerate for 10 minutes to harden before serving.

Nutritional Values per Serving:

Calories: 204

Fat: 17.2g

Protein: 10.2g

Total Carbohydrates: 3g

Dietary Fiber: 0.8g

Net Carbohydrates: 2.2g

Mozzarella Mound Munchies

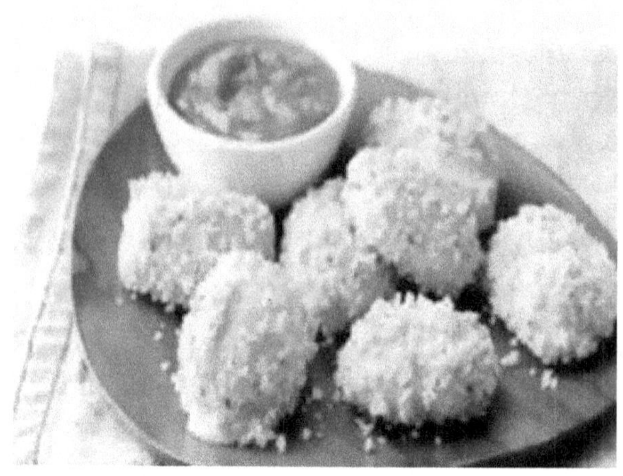

Serves: 3

Prep time: 5 minutes

Cooking Time: 6 minutes

Ingredients:

- ⅓-cup panko bread, herb-flavored

- 2-pcs egg whites

- 6-tbsp mozzarella cheese, molded into 2-tbsp balls

- ¼-cup marinara sauce

Directions:

1. Preheat your oven to 425°F.

2. Toast the panko breadcrumbs for 2 minutes, stirring frequently, in a medium skillet placed over medium heat.

3. Transfer the breadcrumbs in a bowl. Add the egg whites into a separate bowl.

4. Dip a cheeseball into the egg and roll in the panko. Place the breaded cheese on a greased baking sheet, and bake for 3 minutes. Repeat the process for the remaining cheese.

5. Heat the marinara sauce in your microwave oven for half a minute. Serve the breaded cheeseball with the sauce

Nutritional Values per Serving:

Calories: 157

Fat: 13.2g

Protein: 5.9g

Total Carbohydrates: 4.8g

Dietary Fiber: 1.1g

Net Carbohydrates: 3.7g

Philadelphia Potato Praline

Serves:2

Prep time: 30 minutes

Cooking Time: 0 minutes

Ingredients:

- ⅓-cup Philadelphia cream cheese

- 1½-cup coconut, unsweetened and shredded

- 1-tbsp butter

- ¼-tsp ground cinnamon

- Sweetener of choice

Directions:

1. Mix all the ingredients apart from ground cinnamon in a bowl. Refrigerate the mixture and allow setting until it hardens.

2. Divide the mixture into 8 and roll each portion into potato shapes. Place them on a sheet of parchment paper.

3. Sprinkle all over with the cinnamon and store in the fridge for a week before serving.

Nutritional Values per Serving:

Calories: 180

Fat: 15.3g

Protein: 8.9g

Total Carbohydrates: 3.2g

Dietary Fiber: 1.5g

Net Carbohydrates: 1.7g

Tasty Turkey Cheese Cylinders

Serves:1

Prep time: 5 minutes

Cooking Time: 0 minutes

Ingredients:

- 1-oz. turkey, roasted and sliced

- 1-oz. cheese

Directions:

1. Slice the cheese into a long strip, enough to fit the turkey slice.

2. Wrap the turkey slice around the cheese.

Nutritional Values per Serving:

Calories: 162

Fat: 10.9g

Protein: 15.6g

Total Carbohydrates: 3.8g

Dietary Fiber: 0g

Net Carbohydrates: 3.8g

Fried Flaxseed Tortilla Treat

Serves: 3

Prep time: 5 minutes

Cooking Time: 10 minutes

Ingredients:

- 6-shells flaxseed tortillas, sliced into chip-sized cuts

- 3-tbsp olive oil

- A dash of salt and pepper

Directions:

1. Fry the flaxseed chips with olive oil in a large pan placed over medium-high heat. Cook for 10 minutes until the chips become crispy, stirring frequently. Strain the chips and place on a paper towel to drain excess oil.

2. Season with salt and pepper.

Nutritional Values per Serving:

Calories: 36

Fat: 2.8g

Protein: 0.8g

Total Carbohydrates: 2.7g

Dietary Fiber: 0.7g

Net Carbohydrates: 2g

Kingly Kale Crispy Chips

Serves:1

Prep time:4 minutes

Cooking Time: 12 minutes

Ingredients

- 1-bunch large kale, rinsed, drained, and stemless

- 2-tbsp olive oil

- 1-tbsp salt

Directions:

1. Preheat your oven to 350°F.

2. Place the kale in a plastic bag. Pour the oil, and mix well by shaking the bag until coating thoroughly each leaf.

3. Spread the kale onto a baking sheet. Press the leaves flat to obtain an evenly crisped cook for each leaf.

4. Bake for 12 minutes until the edges turn brown while the rest of the kales remain dark green.

5. Sprinkle the salt over the baked kale and serve.

Ambrosial Avocado Puree Pudding

Serves: 3

Prep Time: 5 minutes

Cooking Time: 0 minutes

Ingredients

- 2-ripe Hass avocados, peeled, pitted and cut into chunks

- 2-tsp organic vanilla extract

- 80-drops of liquid sweetener

- 1-can (113.5-oz.) organic coconut milk

- 1-tbsp lime juice from organic lime

Directions

1. Combine all the ingredients in a blender. Blend to a smooth and velvety consistency. Pour the blend equally between three glasses. Chill before serving.

Nutritional Values per Serving:

Calories: 240

Fat: 23.8g

Protein: 2.8g

Total Carbohydrates: 12.8g

Dietary Fiber: 9g

Net Carbohydrates: 3.8g

Power-Packed Butter Balls

Serves: 5

Prep Time: 80 minutes

Cooking Time: 0 minutes

Ingredients:

- 2-tbsp cocoa powder + 1-tbsp for dusting
- 2-tbsp plain oatmeal, gluten-free
- ⅔-cup peanut butter or chia butter
- 1-tbsp organic chia seeds
- 3-tbsp protein powder

Directions:

1. Mix the cocoa powder, oatmeal, peanut butter chia seeds, and protein powder.
2. By using your hand, form balls from the mixture. Dust each ball with cocoa powder.
3. Place the balls in the fridge for 1 hour before serving.

Nutritional Values per Serving:

Calories: 128

Fat: 10.1g

Protein: 4.9g

Total Carbohydrates: 7.2g

Dietary Fiber: 2.9g

Net Carbohydrates: 4.3g

Choco Coco Cups

Serves: 10

Prep Time: 50 minutes

Cooking Time: 0 minutes

Ingredients:

For the Coconut Base:

- ½-cup coconut butter

- ½-cup coconut oil

- ½-cup unsweetened coconut, shredded

- 3-tbsp powdered sweetener

For the Chocolate Topping:

- 3-oz. sugar-free dark chocolate

Directions:

1. Line a muffin pan with 20 mini parchment cups.

2. Heat the coconut butter with the coconut oil in a saucepan placed over low heat. Stir until the butter melts. Stir in the sweetener and coconut and sweetener until fully combined.

3. Divide the mixture equally between the prepared muffin cups. Freeze for 30 minutes until firm.

4. Melt the dark chocolate and spoon over the cold filling. Let it sit for 15 minutes before serving.

Nutritional Values per Serving:

Calories: 240

Fat: 25.3g

Protein: 2.1g

Total Carbohydrates: 5g

Dietary Fiber: 4g

Net Carbohydrates: 1g

Corndog Clumps

Serves: 10

Prep Time: 5 minutes

Cooking Time: 15 minutes

Ingredients:

- ¼-tsp. baking powder

- ¼-tsp. salt

- ½-cup almond flour

- ½-cup flaxseed meal

- 1-tbsp psyllium husk powder

- 3-packets sweetener

- 1-pc large egg

- ⅓-cup sour cream

- ¼-cup melted butter

- ¼-cup coconut milk

- 10-pcs (2-oz.) smoked sausage, sliced in half

Directions:

1. Preheat your oven to 375°F. Grease a 20-cup muffin pan.

2. Combine the first six ingredients in a bowl. Add the egg, sour cream, and butter and mix

well. Pour in the coconut milk, and mix again. Pour the batter in the pan.

3. Insert a sliced sausage into the center of each muffin. Place the pan in the oven.

4. Bake for 12 minutes; thereafter, broil for 3 minutes, set on high heat.

Nutritional Values per Serving:

Calories: 148

Fat: 13.2g

Protein: 3.9g

Total Carbohydrates: 4g

Dietary Fiber: 1.6g

Net Carbohydrates: 3.4g

DESSERTS

Cool Cucumber Sushi with Sriracha Sauce

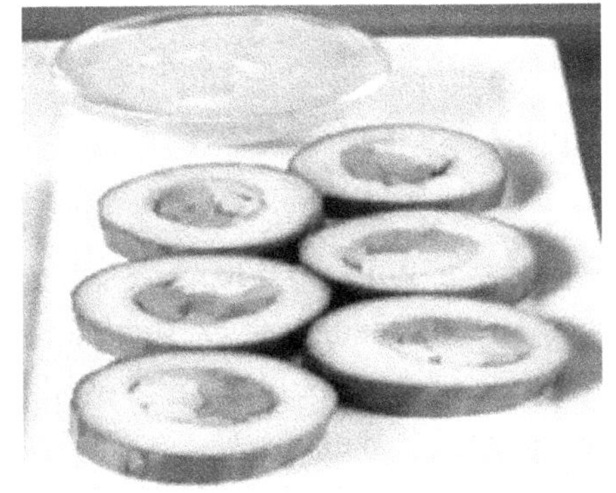

Serves:4

Prep time: 20 minutes

Cooking Time: 0 minutes

Ingredients:

For the Sushi:

- 2-pcs medium cucumbers

- ¼-pc avocado, thinly sliced

- 2-pcs small carrots, thinly sliced

- ½-pc red bell pepper, thinly sliced

- ½-pc yellow bell pepper, thinly sliced

For the Sriracha Sauce:

- ⅓-cup mayonnaise

- 1-tbsp sriracha

- 1-tsp soy sauce, gluten-free

Directions:

1. Slice one end of the cucumbers, and core them by using a small spoon to remove the seeds until completely hollow.

2. By using a butter knife, press the avocado slices into the center of each cucumber. Slide in the carrots and bell peppers until filling up completely each cucumber.

3. To make the dipping sauce, whisk to combine all the sauce ingredients in a bowl.

4. Slice the cucumber into 1"-thick round pieces, Serve with sauce on the side.

Nutritional Values per Serving:

Calories: 110

Fat: 10.1g

Protein: 1.9g

Total Carbohydrates: 4.8g

Dietary Fiber: 2g

Net Carbohydrates: 2.8g

Coco Crack Bake-less Biscuit Bars

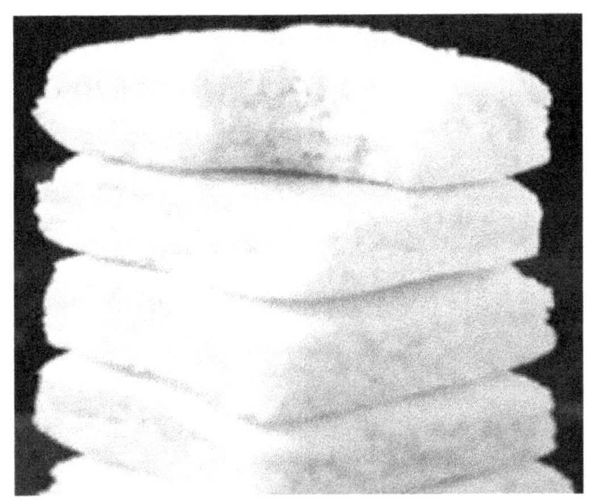

Serves:6

Prep time: 2 minutes

Cooking Time: 3 minutes

Ingredients:

- 3-cups unsweetened coconut flakes, shredded

- 1-cup coconut oil, melted

- ¼-cup liquid sweetener of choice

Directions:

1. Line an 8"-square baking pan with parchment paper. Set aside.

2. Combine all the ingredients in a large mixing bowl. Mix well to a thick batter. (Add a little

liquid sweetener or water if the batter is too crumbly.

3. Pour and press firmly the mixture in the prepared pan. Refrigerate until firm.

4. To serve, slice the hardened mixture into 2" x 8" bars.

Nutritional Values per Serving:

Calories: 106

Fat: 10.5g

Protein: 2.9g

Total Carbohydrates: 2g

Dietary Fiber: 2g

Net Carbohydrates: 0g

Chocolate-Coated Sweet Strawberries

Serves: 8

Prep time:3 hours 5 minutes

Cooking Time: 0 minutes

Ingredients:

- 2-cups melted chocolate chips, dairy-free

- 2-tbsp coconut oil

- 16-pcs fresh strawberries, with stems

Directions:

1. Combine the melted chocolate and coconut oil in a medium bowl. Mix well until fully combined.

2. Scoop the chocolate mixture into each mold of an ice cube tray. Top each with strawberry, with its stem part up. Pour the remaining chocolate mixture over strawberries. Freeze for at least 3 hours until the chocolate hardens.

Nutritional Values per Serving:

Calories: 125

Fat: 11.1g

Protein: 2.7g

Total Carbohydrates: 5g

Dietary Fiber: 1.4g

Net Carbohydrates: 3.6g

Matcha Muffins with Choco-Coco Coating

Serves:4

Prep time: 15 minutes

Cooking Time: 15 minutes

Ingredients:

- ½-cup almond flour

- 1-tbsp yeast

- 1-tbsp cooking matcha powder

- 1-tbsp cashew nuts

- ½-cup milk substitute with hydrogenated vegetable oil

- 1-tbsp peanut butter

- 1-tbsp cacao nibs

- 1-tbsp coconut syrup, gluten-free

- 3-tbsp milk substitute with hydrogenated vegetable oil

- A handful of Goji berries (or blueberries and raspberries) and cocoa nuggets (optional)

Directions:

1. Mix the flour, yeast, matcha powder, cashews. Pour ½-cup of vegetable milk gradually while mixing into the dough.

2. Put the dough in a pre-greased muffin pan. Bake for 15 minutes at 350°F.

3. Mix the peanut butter with cacao, syrup, and milk to make the icing. To serve, pour the icing and garnish with cocoa nuggets and Goji berries.

Nutritional Values per Serving:

Calories: 140

Fat: 10.9g

Protein: 5.1g

Total Carbohydrates: 8.8g

Dietary Fiber: 3.4g

Net Carbohydrates: 5.4g

Cinnamon Cup Cake

Serves: 1

Prep Time: 1 minute

Cooking Time: 0 minutes

Ingredients:

- 1-scoop vanilla protein powder

- ½-tsp baking powder

- 1-tbsp coconut flour

- ½-tsp cinnamon

- 1-tbsp granulated sweetener of choice

- ¼-cup almond milk

- ¼-tsp vanilla extract

- 1-tsp granulated sweetener of choice

- ½-tsp cinnamon powder

For the Butter Glaze:

- 1-tbsp coconut butter, melted

- ½-tsp almond milk

- A pinch of cinnamon powder

Directions:

1. Combine the protein powder, baking powder, coconut flour, cinnamon, and sweetener in a

greased microwave-safe bowl. Mix well until fully combined.

2. Pour the milk, vanilla extract, and sweetener. Mix thoroughly to form a batter. (Add some milk if the batter is too crumbly). Top with a sprinkling of cinnamon powder.

3. Cook in the microwave for 1-minute. Meanwhile, combine all the butter glaze ingredients in a bowl. To serve, top the cake with the butter glaze.

Nutritional Values per Serving:

Calories: 263

Fat: 24.1g

Protein: 7.6g

Total Carbohydrates: 14.2g

Dietary Fiber: 10.3g

Net Carbohydrates: 3.9g

Choco 'Cado Twin Truffles

Serves: 5

Prep Time: 30 minutes

Cooking Time: 0 minutes

Ingredients:

- 1-cup melted dark chocolate chips, dairy-free

- 1-pc small avocado, mashed

- 1-tsp vanilla extract

- ¼-tsp kosher salt

- ¼-cup cocoa powder

Directions:

1. Combine the melted chocolate with avocado, vanilla, and salt in a bowl. Mix well until fully combined. Refrigerate for 20 minutes to firm up slightly.

2. By using a small spoon, scoop about a tablespoon of the chocolate mixture and roll it on the palm of your hand's palm to form a ball. Repeat the process to consume the mixture.

3. Roll each ball in cocoa powder.

Nutritional Values per Serving:

Calories: 68

Fat: 5.8g

Protein: 1.6g

Total Carbohydrates: 4.2g

Dietary Fiber: 1.8g

Net Carbohydrates: 2.4g

Butter Ball Bombs

Serves: 10

Prep Time: 65mins

Cooking Time: 0 minutes

Ingredients:

- 8-tbsp (1 stick) butter, softened to room temperature

- ⅓-cup sweetener

- ½-teaspoon. pure vanilla extract

- ½-teaspoon. kosher salt

- 2-cups almond flour

- ⅔-cup unsweetened dark chocolate chips, dairy-free

Directions:

1. Use your hand mixer and beat the butter in a large bowl until light and fluffy. Add the vanilla extract, sweetener, and salt. Beat again until fully combined.

2. Add gradually the almond flour, beating continuously until no dry portions remain. Fold in the chocolate chips. Cover the bowl with a plastic wrap and refrigerate for 20 minutes to firm slightly.

3. By using a small spoon, scoop the dough to form into small balls.

Nutritional Values per Serving:

Calories: 51

Fat: 4.3g

Protein: 0.7g

Total Carbohydrates: 2.7g

Dietary Fiber: 0.4g

Net Carbohydrates: 2.3g

Choco Coco Cookies

Serves: 6

Prep Time: 10 minutes

Cooking Time: 15 minutes

Ingredients:

- ¼-cup coconut oil

- 4-pcs egg yolks

- 2-tablespoon sweetener

- 1-cup dark unsweetened chocolate chips

- 1-cup coconut flakes

- 4-tablespoon butter, softened

- ¾-cup walnuts,choppedroughly

Directions:

1. Preheat your oven to 350°F. Use a parchment paper to line a baking tray.

2. Mix all the ingredients in a large mixing bowluntil fully combined.

3. Form cookies out of the mixture, and place them in the baking tray. Bake for 15 minutes until golden.

4. Serve and enjoy.

Nutritional Values per Serving:

Calories: 130

Fat: 11.5g

Protein: 2.9g

Total Carbohydrates: 6g

Dietary Fiber: 2.2g

Net Carbohydrates: 3.8g

Carrot Compact Cake

Serves: 8

Prep Time: 20 minutes

Cooking Time: 0 minutes

Ingredients:

- 1-block (8-oz.) cream cheese, softened

- ¾-cup coconut flour

- 1-teaspoon sweetener

- ½-teaspoon pure vanilla extract

- 1-teaspoon cinnamon

- ¼-teaspoon ground nutmeg

- 1-cup carrots, grated

- 1-cup unsweetened coconut, shredded

- ½-cup pecans, chopped

Directions:

1. Mix the first six ingredients in a large mixing bowl. Mix well by using a hand mixer until fully combined. Fold in the pecans and carrots.

2. Form 16 balls from the mixture, and roll each ball in shredded coconut.

Nutritional Values per Serving:

Calories: 94

Fat: 8.3g

Protein: 2.8g

Total Carbohydrates: 5.2g

Dietary Fiber: 3.1g

Net Carbohydrates: 2.1g

Chilled Cream

Serves: 8

Prep Time: 8 hours 15 minutes

Cooking Time: 0 minutes

Ingredients:

- 2-cans (15-oz.) coconut milk, refrigerated for at least 3 hours

- 2-cups heavy cream

- 1-teaspoon pure vanilla extract

- ¼-cup sweetener

- A pinch of kosher salt

Directions:

1. Spoon the refrigerated coconut milk into a large bowl. Leave the liquid in the can. By using a hand mixer, beat the milk until turning creamy. Set aside.

2. Beat the heavy cream in a separate large bowl until it forms soft peaks. Add the vanilla and sweetener. Beat again until fully combined.

3. Fold in the whipped milk into the whipped cream. Mix well and transfer the mixture in a loaf pan.

4. Place the pan in the freezer for 5 hours until the mixture becomes solid.

Nutritional Values per Serving:

Calories: 340

Fat: 34.8g

Protein: 3.7g

Total Carbohydrates: 5.2g

Dietary Fiber: 2.1g

Net Carbohydrates: 3.1g

AUTOPHAGY

The human body contains many intricate regulatory mechanisms that ensure the normal functioning of millions of cells. One such regulatory mechanism is known as autophagy. Autophagy plays a significant role in the body as it ensures the removal of old, worn-out substances, including damaged organelles, abnormal or old proteins, and cell debris. It is essentially a recycling process that occurs in all eukaryotes. It is also involved in the regulation of a variety of cellular functions, such as cell death, cell differentiation and growth, oxidative stress, the nutrient-deficiency stress response and organelle turnover.

Autophagy is a highly conserved process and is a major reliever of various stress conditions for cells. It also plays an essential role in the extension of a cell's lifespan. The term autophagy was coined by Christian de Duve about half a century ago. Since then, it has been the focus of many types of research and has helped us understand the physiological processes of cell regulation and recycling in the body.

Significance of Autophagy

Autophagy is a hallmark of energy generation processes when the cell's energy reserves are scarce and the body is in the starvation phase. The breakdown of cellular components provides energy for metabolic processes which primarily include the production of new proteins and membranes. It also provides the necessary energy for survival in stressful conditions such as starvation and nutrient deficiency. Autophagy is the main process that maintains the health of cells and organs as it replaces old and outdated components of a cell with new ones.

Autophagy affects the overall metabolic homeostasis of the body; nearly all the vital metabolic processes that occur in the body are directly or indirectly dependent on this process to function optimally. Furthermore, autophagy also plays a diverse role in the functioning of the immune system.

Types of Autophagy

There are two main types of autophagy: non-selective and selective autophagy. Selective autophagy occurs under normal conditions for the purpose of renewal and recycling of cellular components. It targets a specific substrate that needs to be removed from the cell, including damaged mitochondria, aggregates of abnormal proteins and different types of pathogens. These processes allow the removal of damaged organelles from the cell to ease the unwanted cellular burden and help to maintain the steady-state turnover of the organelles.

Selective autophagy can be further classified into different types depending on the organelle being targeted for degradation. For instance, the degradation of peroxisomes is termed pexophagy and autophagy of the mitochondria is termed mitophagy.

Non-selective autophagy occurs in cellular stress conditions, primarily when the cell faces nutrient deficiency and starvation. It does not target any specific organelle or substance and instead catabolizes random cellular components to meet the energy needs of the cell.

Melany Flores

THE SCIENCE BEHIND AUTOPHAGY

Autophagy is a complex degradative process that involves many proteins and various pathways. Generally, this self-cannibalization mechanism is comprised of the formation of a specialized vesicle that contains abnormal and long-lived proteins and organelles in its cytoplasm. This vesicle then fuses with lysosomes that carry out the degradation process.

In this way, the cell can capture its own organelles and consume them by degrading them in the lysosome. The various benefits of autophagy have significantly increased its importance in research and studies all over the world.

Types of Autophagy According to Mechanism

Autophagy is a complex process, and it varies according to the needs of the cell and the size of the products to be degraded. Depending on the mechanism used for the transfer of organelles (cargo) to the lysosome, there are three main types of autophagy mechanisms. These include:

- Macro-autophagy

- Micro-autophagy

- Chaperone-mediated autophagy (CMA)

The mechanism of microautophagy and macroautophagy is somewhat similar as both are comprised of the dynamic rearrangement of the membrane to enclose the cytoplasm and the cargo that needs to be degraded. However, while microautophagy involves the simple engulfment of cargo at the surfaces of the lysosome by invagination and septation of the membrane of the lysosome, macroautophagy is dependent on the formation of a specialized double membraned vesicle around the cargo (the autophagosome) via *de novo* synthesis of the membrane. The autophagosome then fuses with a lysosome and empties the inner contents into the lysosome for degradation. In both cases, the membrane-bound content is degraded, and the resulting nutrients and macromolecules are transported back into the cytosol to be utilized for various metabolic processes.

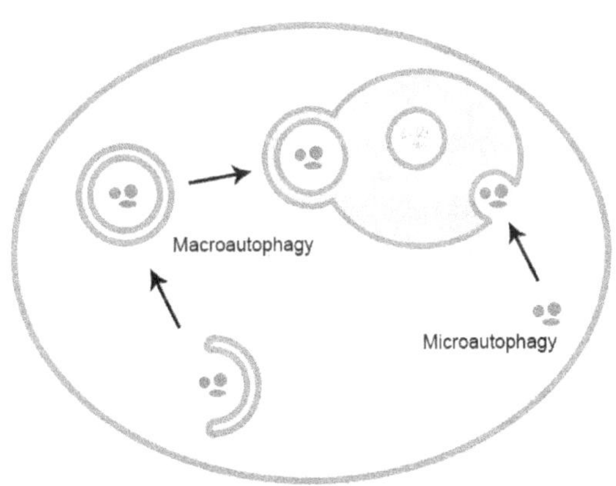

Figure 1. Types of autophagy.

The third type of autophagy does not involve any special membrane arrangements or the formation of a vesicle. Instead, it uses specific chaperones that directly transfer abnormally formed proteins and other cargo across the membrane of lysosome for degradation.

The most common and most widely understood autophagy is macroautophagy. Most published studies have focused on macroautophagy; this book will also be focusing on macroautophagy to avoid confusion and help us better understand the process and its effects on our body.

Mechanism of Macroautophagy

Autophagy involves the formation of a specific cavity or vesicle that engulfs or surround the substances that need to be degraded. This membrane-bound structure then fuses with the lysosome and transfer its contents, termed as cargo, into it for degradation. This process involves the role of around 16 different proteins that ensure the proper execution of autophagy. The complete process of autophagy can be divided into seven distinct steps. These are given below:

- Induction

- Nucleation

- Expansion and recognition of cargo

- Recycling of proteins

- Fusion of vesicle with the lysosome

- Digestion

- Recycling of cargo

Formation of Autophagosome

The primary step in the process of autophagy is the production of autophagosome or the vesicle. Around sixteen different Atg proteins control the formation of the autophagosome. The average diameter of the autophagosome is approximately 0.9 μm in yeast and about 1.5 μm in mammals. Various environmental cues, such as nutrient deficiency, are picked up by cell receptors such as mTORC1 that become inactive and cause the activation of the ULK1 complex that then affects the activity of P13K complex. This complex plays a central role in the early stages of the formation of the autophagosome by mediating the production of the phagophore from which the isolation membrane of autophagosome originates. Various Atg proteins including Atg-12, Atg-9, Atg-5 and Atg16L1 play a critical role in the elongation of isolation membrane.

In the next step, the autophagosome fuses with the cell vesicles (derived from the endosome) and forms a structure known as amphisome. This structure combines with the lysosome to form the autolysosome. When the components of the autophagosome are transferred to the lysosome, they are attacked by hydrolases and degraded into smaller molecules. These molecules help to replenish the energy and metabolic needs of the body, and the signal of the presence of a high level of nutrients reactivate the mTORC1 that leads to the suppression of autophagy.

Stepwise Process of Autophagy

The primary step in the process of autophagy, where the production of autophagosome occurs, is termed as induction or initiation. In this step, the membrane of the cell begins to expand and forms the phagophore, which is a double membrane sequestering compartment. This membrane expands to form the spherical autophagosome and wraps itself around the cargo. At this stage, the LC3-II is cleaved from the outer part of this double-membraned structure. The autophagosome then finds the lysosome, and its outer membrane fuses with the lysosomal membrane to form a structure known as the autolysosome.

However, in some cases, the autophagosome fuses with an endosome and forms a specialized structure known as the amphisome before it reaches and fuses with a lysosome.

The cargo is delivered from the autophagosome to the lysosome and is degraded and exported back into the cytoplasm through lysosomal channels known as permeases. The products of autophagy are reused for various processes in the cell.

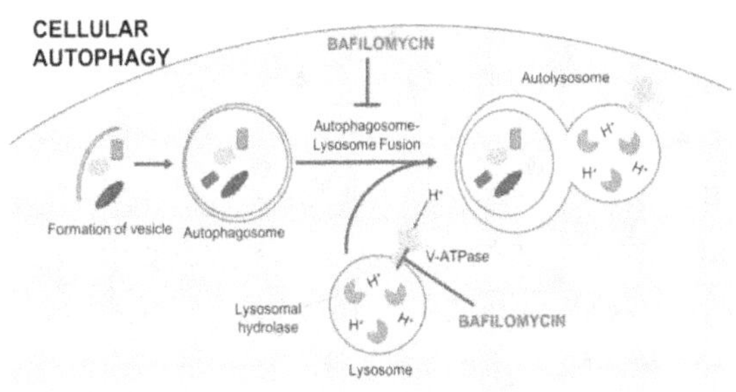

Figure 2. Formation of autophagosome.

Genetics of Autophagy

Several genome-wide studies have highlighted the role of various genes in the process of autophagy. These autophagy-related genes are marked as ATG genes and are involved in multiple cellular processes of autophagy. These genes were initially identified in yeast, and various studies suggest that there is conservation of autophagy machinery among all eukaryotes. Various orthologs of ATG genes of yeast have also been found to be present in various higher organisms.

In yeast, the induction of the autophagosome is regulated by the Atg1-Atg13-Atg17-Atg31-Atg29 kinase complex. In mammals, the autophagosome is formed by a homolog of Atg1 ULK1 or ULK2,

Atg13, RB1-inducible coiled-coil 1 (RB1CC1/FIP200) and C12orf44/ATG101. This complex (ULK1/2-ATG13-RB1CC1) will carry out autophagy regardless of the nutrient status of the cells.

Autophagy and the Nobel Prize-Winning Experiment

After many years of studies and research, the mechanism of autophagy was understood only recently. Yoshinori Ohsumi was given the Nobel Prize in Physiology and Medicine in 2016 for his successful experiment that highlighted the mechanism of autophagy in yeast cells.

KEY REGULATORS OF AUTOPHAGY

Autophagy is a naturally occurring process in the body that is primarily induced in response to various environmental and physiological stress factors. Some environmental factors are deprivation of food, deprivation of oxygen and exposure to high temperatures. The most significant physiological factor of induction of autophagy is aging. Moreover, the relationship between autophagy and aging also shares a remarkable interaction at the molecular level.

Nutrient homeostasis maintains the physiological functions of the cells. Autophagy is a highly efficient process that carries out the recycling of the nutrients in the body and thus maintains the nutrient homeostasis. The process of autophagy is activated when cells undergo nutritional stress, which include nutrient deficiency (starvation) or nutrient excess. Two protein kinases, AMP-activated protein kinase and the mammalian target of rapamycin (mTOR), regulate the process of autophagy. These enzymes monitor the energy and amino acids levels in the cell. When autophagy is activated in starvation conditions, the damaged organelles and proteins are degraded and the nutrient status of the cell is replenished. However, uncontrolled or unnecessary induction of autophagy can lead to cell death. Thus, the equilibrium between the induction and suppression of autophagy is crucial for determining the fate of the cell. Nutrient excess can also lead to autophagy.

There are three main kinases that carry out the regulation of macroautophagy at the cellular level. These kinases act as sensors and read the environmental and physiological signals that lead to the induction of autophagy. They include AMP-activated protein kinases (AMPK), mechanistic target of rapamycin complex1 (MTORC1) and cAMP- activated protein kinase (PKA).

Relationship Between Autophagy, Cellular Energy Levels, and Starvation

In the 1970s, various researchers established a definite relationship between the nutritional status of a cell and autophagy. Starvation was identified as the first stimulus that led to the activation of autophagy. The benefits of the process of autophagy in starved cells were quite clear as it played a central role in the energy homeostasis of the cell by recycling cellular components and amino acids through catabolic action of lysosomes.

Autophagy carries out catabolism of different essential nutrients of the diet. When there is a depletion of nutrients, autophagy ensures the survival of the cell by carrying out the degradation of intracellular proteins to provide essential amino acids. These amino acids can be used in the synthesis of proteins or can directly enter the Krebs's cycle for the generation of energy currency, i.e., ATP. The presence of nutrients and the replenishing of cellular energy levels lead to the suppression of autophagy. In this way, autophagy is a self-regulated process which is highly sensitive to the energy markers of the cells.

Another role of autophagy in the maintenance of energy levels and nutrient pools of the cell is that it functions to mobilize the intracellular lipid stores and glycogen reserves to generate energy during the period of starvation. The breakdown of intracellular stores of nutrients by macroautophagy can also occur when there are high levels of glucose and fats in the cells. This mechanism helps the cell to manage the size of intracellular stores and avoids nutrient burdening of the cell.

There are special nutrient sensors that help medicate the process of autophagy in the cell. These sensors provide the required communication between the nutritional status of the cell and autophagy. The essential mammalian sensor of nutritional status that also regulates the process of macroautophagy is the mammalian target of rapamycin (mTOR). These enzymes read nutritional cues such as the presence of amino acids, ATP levels, and insulin in the body and upregulate or downregulate the process of autophagy accordingly.

Starvation that is primarily marked by reduced levels of nutrients and insulin in the body that leads to the inactivation of mTOR through the influence of AMP-activated protein kinase (AMPK) is another cellular nutrient sensor. Inactivation of mTOR leads to the production of the autophagy initiation complex and the formation of autophagosomes.

WHAT CAN GO WRONG WITH AUTOPHAGY?

Autophagy is the double-edged sword in the human body.

Autophagy is a highly regulated process, and its degradative abilities make its regulation an essential entity. Any kind of errors and mutations in the genes or proteins involved in this pathway can have deleterious effects on the cells. Defects in autophagy have been found to be linked with various diseases and disorders, and this indicates the physiological significance of this process in the body. These processes include cellular differentiation, homeostasis, growth and development, and starvation.

Various studies have identified mutations in the ATG genes to be the underlying cause of multiple diseases in human, which include infectious diseases, neurodegenerative diseases and different types of cancers.

A list of diseases and their associated mutation in ATG and other genes related to autophagy are given in Table 1.

Table 1. The link between various autophagy-related genetic disorders and diseases

Sr #	Stage in Autophagy process	Gene Involved	Disease in Humans
1	Formation of autophagosome	ATG16L1	Crohn's disease
2	Formation of autophagosome	ATG5	Asthma and Lupus
3	Formation of autophagosome	EI24/PIG8	Breast Cancer
4	Formation of autophagosome	BECN1	Prostate, ovarian and colorectal cancer
5	Maturation of autophagosome	SPG15	Hereditary spastic paraparesis type 15
6	Induction of mitophagy (autophagy of mitochondria)	PARK6/PINK1	Parkinson's disease

Apart from genetic defects, malfunctioning of autophagy can have deleterious effects on the body. These include various kinds of cancer, muscular disorders, liver disease, neurodegeneration and recurrent pathogenic infections. Therefore, autophagy is a double-edged sword that can benefit or harm the cell in different conditions. The beneficial and harmful role of autophagy in the human body and how it can act in both ways is summarized in **Table 2**.

Table 2. The positive and negative effects of autophagy in the body

Disease	Positive effects of autophagy	Negative effects of autophagy
Cancer	Functions as a tumor suppressor and removes damaged organelles that could generate free radicals and increase	Promotes the survival of cancer cells inside a tumor where there is deficiency of nutrients. It can protect the cancer cells from cell death, and hinders

	chances of mutations	chemotherapeutic methods
Liver disease	Removes damaged endoplasmic reticulum	Excessive mitochondrial autophagy can lead to tissue damage
Muscular disorder	Decreases the effects of lysosomal disease	Increased autophagy and accumulation of autophagosomes leads to defects in cell function
Neurodegeneration	Removes toxic aggregates of protein	May triggerdeath of neurons that carry aggregated proteins
Pathogen infection	Provides protection against viruses and bacteria	Can allow pathogens to survive and grow, and provides nutrients for their growth

Role of Autophagy in Various Diseases

Autophagy and Cancer

Abnormal growth and death of cells are the hallmarks of cancer. This feature suggests a specific role of autophagy-related proteins in the triggering and progression of cancer. Autophagy keeps a check in the abnormality of components of the cell and can be considered to be a quality control center. The failure of the process of autophagy can lead to the unsuccessful degradation and removal of abnormal cells that can lead to carcinogenesis.

Various ATG genes, including the ATG5, ATG2, ATG12 ABD and UVRAG genes, have been found to be linked with several types of cancers and have been affected with microsatellite instability and point mutations. The relationship between autophagy and cancer has been an area of interest and many oncology-related studies are now focusing on the therapeutic role of the autophagy-related gene in cancer.

The autophagy gene Beclin-1 that is involved in the early stages of autophagosome formation is a tumor suppressor gene. Autophagy can kill tumor cells by removing damaged mitochondria and other abnormal organelles. Similarly, PTEN and p53 are bona fide tumor suppressor genes that can also induce autophagy in the cells. Thus, autophagy has a protective effect against cancer progression as it promotes the growth of healthy cells and destroys the abnormal cancerous cells.

Autophagy and Neurodegenerative Diseases

Various single-gene mutations linked with many multisystem disorders in children have been found to be reported in autophagy genes. These inborn errors in the autophagy system predominantly affect the health and development of the central nervous system. They have been associated with causing epilepsy, malformation of the brain, intellectual disability delay in development, neurodegeneration, and disorder of movement.

These mutations affect the various stages of autophagy and lead to a wide class of disorders termed as congenital disorders of autophagy that are part of another diverse group of disorders known as inborn errors of metabolism.

Autophagy and Inflammatory disease

There is emerging evidence that defects in autophagy play an essential role in the triggering and progression of various acute and chronic inflammatory diseases. These include Crohn's disease, pulmonary hypertension, infectious diseases, inflammatory bowel disease, cystic fibrosis, lupus, and diabetes. Autophagy impacts the regulation of various inflammatory diseases by several mechanisms. These include:

- A xenophagic response initiated by autophagy where it directly participates in the clearance of bacteria by capturing and delivering the bacteria to the lysosome for degradation.

- Autophagic assists in antigen presentation by digesting the invading pathogens.

- Various proteins involved in autophagy play an essential role in controlling many proinflammatory responses, such as the production of proinflammatory cytokines and the maintenance of the quality of mitochondrial function.

- Autophagic degradation of toxic aggregates of proteins plays a protective role in tissues. Otherwise, serious diseases such as cystic fibrosis can occur.

Melany Flores

Role of Autophagy in Inflammation and Related Diseases

Autophagy is a multidimensional process and the association between autophagy and the inflammatory response of the body is rather complex. There are various studies that suggest that autophagy controls the development and survival of the inflammatory machinery and thus orchestrates the inflammatory response. The cells of the inflammatory machinery that are directly regulated by the process of autophagy include lymphocytes, neutrophils, and macrophages. These cells are involved in the development as well as pathogenesis of inflammation in tissues and organs. Recent evidence indicates that autophagy plays a critical role in acute and chronic inflammatory processes. This role potentially impacts the pathogenesis and progression of various inflammatory diseases.

Macrophages

Macrophages are a significant part of our defense system and can destroy pathogens by producing inflammatory cytokines, or by uptake and intracellular destruction. There is growing evidence that suggests that upregulation of autophagy leads to increased killing of ingested pathogens in macrophages. Mice with defective autophagy systems in neutrophils and macrophages tend to be more prone to infections from intracellular pathogens such as *L. monocytogenes* and *T. gondii.*

Autophagy also acts as a regulator of inflammatory process by keeping the population of macrophages in the body in check. It has been reported that autophagy is induced in several activated macrophages when exposed to oxidative stress in the form of reactive oxygen species (ROS) causing an increase in autophagosomes that lead to the death and removal of these macrophages. This can be helpful in controlling the level of inflammation in the tissues.

Neutrophils

Neutrophils are multifunctional cells of the immune system. They play a central role in the innate immune system. The presence of inflammation in tissues recruits neutrophils to the site of infection. Neutrophils then engulf the microorganism and render it inactive by fusing it with phagosomes, resulting in the formation of phagolysosomes. Inside the phagolysosomes, the action of ROS and antimicrobial peptides lead to the destruction and clearance of pathogens. The apoptosis of neutrophils leads to a decrease in inflammation. Autophagy occurs in neutrophils in both phagocytosis-dependent and independent manners. The most widely studied function of autophagy involves its role in neutrophil death, which governs the level of inflammation in the body.

Lymphocytes

Autophagy plays an important role in both innate and adaptive immune responses. These immune responses include the homeostasis of the immune system and presentation of antigens. There exists a complex and crucial relationship between T lymphocytes and autophagy. The activation of the T cell receptor (TCR) is a strong trigger for autophagy in T lymphocytes. Several autophagy-related genes are involved in the proliferation of T cells. It has been found that T lymphocytes with defective Atg3, Atg5 and Atg7 genes have decreased proliferation rates and increased rates of cell death. Autophagy plays an important role in the homeostasis of T cells; it mediates the selection of thymocytes (lymphocytes that are present in the thymus gland) and regulates their functions. Autophagic defects in thymocytes have been linked with various autoimmune diseases. Moreover, absence of autophagy leads to the accumulation of toxic reactive oxygen species in the lymphocytes which can lead to various physiological complications. The Beclin-1 gene has been found to be involved in the development of lymphocytes and proves that a critical relationship exists between autophagy and apoptosis.

Autophagy has a direct role in mediating antigen presentation to antigen-specific T cells. This process is crucial for the induction of the acquired immune response in the body. The molecules of MHC class II have been found to localize on autophagosomes. The presentation of antigens, both viral and self, by MHC class II molecules to antigen-specific CD4+ T cells is regulated by autophagic machinery. When the body is infected with a certain virus, for instance, the human simplex virus 1, the autophagic machinery regulates the MHC class I-dependent presentation of viral antigens to CD8+ T cells.

Apart from T lymphocytes, the Atg5 gene has been found to be crucial for the growth and development of B lymphocytes. Various studies suggest that Atg5 genes play an important role in the certain differentiation stages of B cells.

Crohn's Disease

Crohn's disease (CD) is a chronic disease that affects the bowel. It is characterized by inflammation, ulceration, and neutrophil influx in the upper layer of the intestine. Various environmental and genetic factors have been linked with CD. Recent studies have also found links between CD and genes that are associated with autophagy. These genes include ATG16L, and NOD2. The NOD2 protein functions as an intracellular sensor or detector of bacteria. It has the ability to induce autophagy in the intestinal cells when detecting peptidoglycan present in bacterial cell walls. Various studies in humans suggest that three NOD2 variants are associated with CD. These variants lead to loss of function of NOD2 and may contribute to the pathogenesis of CD. Moreover, a variant of the ATG16lL gene, which is involved in the synthesis of autophagosome formation, has been found to be a major risk factor for CD.

Infectious Disease

Autophagy plays a crucial role in the immune system as it can exert various anti-pathogen and anti-bacterial functions. These features tend to impart beneficial features to the autophagic process in various infectious diseases.

For instance, in the case of a *Mycobacterium tuberculosis* infection, the autophagy pathway plays a crucial role in rendering resistance against various bacterial, viral and protozoan infections. Mycobacterium tuberculosis is an intracellular parasite and dwells within cells. It can survive within phagosomes by interfering with the synthesis of phagolysosome. By promoting autophagy, the cell can get rid of the pathogen and can provide protection for the body from various infections. The role of autophagy in providing defense against other microbial pathogens including *Legionella pneumophila* and *Shigella* has also been reported.

Pulmonary Hypertension

Pulmonary arterial hypertension (PAH) is a complex disease. It is characterized by vasoconstriction, the thickening of the artery, and increase in pulmonary artery pressure. The decrease in oxygen levels in the lungs lead to the induction of autophagy which lead to damage and fibrosis of the artery.

Cystic Fibrosis

Cystic fibrosis (CF) is a disease of lungs and airways and is characterized by an inflammation of airways, accumulation of mucous in the airways, and absence of mucociliary clearance, primarily due to the mutation of a certain protein termed as cystic fibrosis transmembrane conductance regulator (CFTR).

It has been recently found that the mutation in the CFTR gene is linked with an abnormal autophagic response. The CFTR defect and autophagy deficiency together lead to the accumulation of aggregates of protein in the pulmonary tissues and inflammation of the lung.

Chronic Obstructive Pulmonary Disease

Chronic obstructive pulmonary disease (COPD) is a lung disease characterized by chronic airway inflammation and lung damage. Macroautophagy plays a complex role in the pathogenesis of COPD. Elevated levels of the LC3b-II protein have been found in blood samples of COPD patients when compared with non-COPD controls. The level of LC3b-II correlates to the over function of autophagy in the lung cells.

Genetic mutations in two macroautophagy pathway members, Beclin-1 and LC3b, have been found to be associated with a reduction in the rate of cell death in lung cells which are exposed to cigarette smoke. Furthermore, there was an inhibition of macroautophagic flux in macrophages from COPD tissues, which may contribute to inflammation in lungs and air passages.

Other systemic inflammatory diseases

There are other systemic inflammatory diseases that have been found to be associated with autophagic defects. For instance, studies show that polymorphisms in the autophagy gene Atg5can lead to increased susceptibility of systemic lupus erythematosus (SLE). SLE is a heterogenous disease caused by an autoimmune response that targets the self-antigens of the dying cells. This anomaly results in the destruction of tissues and organs by our own immune system and the driving force behind it is the defective autophagy process. Other defects in autophagy have been linked to several inflammation-associated metabolic disorders including obesity and diabetes.

Melany Flores

THE ROLE OF AUTOPHAGY IN CANCER

Autophagy playsa dual role in cancer biology as it can regulate cancer promotion and suppression. This dual role highlights the importance of autophagy in the body and categorizes it as a double-edged sword of human physiology. Under certain physiological conditions, autophagy acts as a tumor suppressor and protects the cell from the progression and survival of cancerous cells. Under different physiological conditions, autophagy helps to promote the progression and growth of cancer cells and protects them from apoptosis. Due to this, some anticancer drugs that directly regulate autophagy have been developed. Such autophagy-based chemotherapy can be used in cancer-cell destruction or survival.

It is known that autophagy regulation in the body influences the expression of tumor promotor genes (oncogenes) or tumor suppressor proteins. The factors that are involved in the suppression of tumors are negatively regulated by mTOR and AMPK. This leads to the induction of autophagy and suppresses the initiation of cancer. On the other hand, oncogenes are activated by mTOR and AKT, which is associated with the suppression of autophagy and promotes the progression of cancer. In this way, the underlying pathways that regulate autophagy indirectly decide the fate of cancerous cells in the body.

Autophagy also plays a direct role in the promotion of cancer. Abnormal autophagy processes lead to a decrease in the degradation of old and damaged organelles and proteins in cells with increased oxidative stress. This leads to the development of cancer.

Primarily, the basal process of autophagy suppresses cancer. The mutation of autophagic proteins lead to an increased risk of various types of cancers. For instance, BIF-1 proteins that are associated with BECN1 have been found to be anomalous in colorectal and stomach cancer. Similarly, the UVRAG proteins that are associated with BECN1 function as a major regulator of autophagy, and the presence of mutated UVRAG leads to a reduction in the process of autophagy, resulting inan increased proliferation rate of colorectal cancer cells.

Conversely, the tumor promoter rule of autophagy highlights the fact that high cellular levels of autophagy are linked with different types of RAS-activated cancers including pancreatic cancers. This implies that methods to suppress autophagy lead to a decrease in the proliferation of cancerous cells which improves tumor suppression.

Hence, autophagy regulates tumor initiation and suppression. The diverse roles of autophagy as an inducer of cancer and as a tumor suppressor are discussed in the sections below and summarized in Table

Autophagy as a Regulator of Tumor Suppression

The intrinsic ability of autophagy to remove abnormal proteins and to degrade dysfunctional organelles and maintain the cellular homeostasis makes it a diehard tumor suppressor. The presence of any kind of mutation in autophagic genes or any metabolic error related to the physiological function of autophagy results in deleterious effects on the cell. These effects may manifest themselves in form of various metabolic disorders and cancers of various parts including the ovaries, breasts and prostate.

Various studies suggest that the autophagy mutation of the BECN gene that encodes Beclin-1, which is an important part of autophagic machinery, can appear clinically in various forms of cancer. Beclin-1 is a tumor suppressor gene as it promotes the autophagy process by the synthesis of autophagosomes. Mutations in this gene lead to increased proliferation of cancer cells as the process of autophagy that keeps a check on the cellular quality has become compromised. A decrease in cellular Beclin-1 level has also been observed in cases of other cancers, including cervical squamous-cell carcinomas and hepatocellular cancers.

There is experimental evidence that suggests that the mutation of certain other autophagic genes can also lead to tumor suppression. Certain proteins, such as UV radiation resistance-associated gene (UVRAG) function as tumor suppressor genes. Under normal conditions, it acts as a positive regulator of autophagy. The decrease in UVRAG causes an impaired autophagosome development and a decreased level of cellular autophagy. This results in an increase in cancer cell proliferation of different types of cancers, including colon, stomach, breast, and prostate cancers.

Knockout studies involving core autophagic proteins have been carried out to study the cancer-suppression role of autophagy in mice. It was found that the knockout of ATG5 and ATG7 genes from hepatocytes resulted in liver cancers. The reason behind the appearance of this major pathology was that the liver cells were unable to clear themselves from damaged mitochondria and protect themselves from oxidative stress. Autophagy prevents the cell from tumor generation by regulating the levels of reactive oxygen species (ROS). Mitochondrial damage produces excessive ROS, which is one of the major triggers of carcinogenesis. Autophagy functions to protect the cell from various stresses, and impaired autophagy has catastrophic effects on cell function and quality, and they then progress as defective cancerous cells. Similar results have been obtained by studying cell lines that are deficient of autophagic regulators, such as ATG3, ATG5 and ATG9. These findings highlight the critical role of autophagy in tumor suppression; impaired autophagy can therefore lead to oncogenesis.

Autophagy as a Regulators of Tumor Promotion

The other role of autophagy in cancer is of tumor promotion. Various studies indicate that the process of autophagy promotes the survival of cancer cells and aids in the progression of tumors in later or advanced stages of cancer. So, autophagy acts as a tumor suppressor and tries to stop the progression of cancer in early stages, but if it fails due to any reason and the cancer spreads and reaches the metastasis stage, autophagy aids the tumor cells in surviving and developing.

The cells inside tumors suffer from various stresses, including low oxygen levels and poor availability of nutrients. Autophagy plays an intrinsic role in aiding the tumor cells in surviving these stresses. It also leads to the activation of autophagy in the central part of tumors where cells are exposed to extreme hypoxic conditions. The decrease in cellular autophagy due to the deletion of

Beclin-1 increases cell death in tumors as the hypoxic and nutrient deficient cells are no longer protected by autophagy.

In addition to providing protection against the oxidative stresses of tumor cells, autophagy provides energy to proliferating tumors. It carries out the recycling of intracellular organelles and components and fulfills the metabolic needs of the growing tumor cells.

In animal models with impaired autophagy processes, tumor cells have been observed to undergo metabolic stress which leads to the decreased survival of cancer cells. In this way, autophagy plays a central role in the survival of tumor cells by improving their stress tolerance and by supplying the cells with necessary nutrients to meet their metabolic demands. Without these tumor-protective effects of autophagy as observed in knockout or knockdown animal models of autophagy, there is an increased rate of tumor cell death.

Table 3. Dual role of autophagy in cancer

Sr #	Autophagy induction under stress conditions in cancer cells	
	Tumor Suppressor Effects	*Tumor Promotor Effects*
1	Inhibits the growth of the tumor	Aids tumor cells to overcome various stresses
2	Maintains the homeostasis of the cell	Provides tumor cells with the required metabolic energy
3	Provides protection against cellular stresses	Degrades damaged organelles
4	Decreases the formation of tumor	Favors the formation of tumor by not removing oxidative stress

AUTOPHAGY AND ITS ROLE IN AGING

Autophagy is the renewal system of the cell. The more efficient the system is, the more replenished and rejuvenated the cells and organs become. This effect of autophagy on the revitalization of the human system suggests its direct role in human aging. Various studies have found that there is a definite genetic link between the genes of autophagy and the aging process.

There is a decrease in the efficiency of autophagy with age, and these findings have been extensively investigated in the yeast system. Mutants that carry defects in macroautophagy related genes have a shorter lifespan as compared to control organisms. Similarly, in nematodes,for example *Caenorhabditis elegans*, the mutants carrying a loss of function mutation in Atg1, Atg7 and Beclin-1 showed a significant decrease in their lifespan as compared to normal samples. The knockout studies of autophagy-related genes in other organisms, including fruit fly and murine models highlight the importance of the autophagy process in aging and allowing for longer lifespans.

As mentioned before, autophagy is the quality control center of the body. As we age, autophagy loses its efficiency, and there is a progressive loss in the quality of organs function – this is also the primary indication of aging. As the function of autophagy wanes off, various age-associated pathologies start to manifest themselves. The accumulation of different toxic and abnormal organelles and proteins in the cell further aid the triggering of age-related problems, such as a reduction in muscle mass, cardiac malfunction, accumulation of lipids and cholesterol, memory loss and neurodegeneration and insulin insensitivity.

Certain other factors related to autophagy also play a vital role in the process of aging. For instance, there is a loss of genomic maintenance by autophagy due to the aging process. Oxidative stress that can harm the DNA structure and its integrity is significantly reduced by autophagic actions, and various studies also suggest that there is a definitive role of autophagy in cell cycle progression and in DNA repair systems. All these processes ensure the genomic maintenance that is equivalent to an error-free, high-functioning genome as present in a young individual. This genomic maintenance is gradually lost with aging.

Autophagy Immunosenescence and Aging

As we age, there is a gradual decrease in the activity of autophagic processes, it even becomes defective in elder humans. For instance, in old livers, the efficiency of glucagon metabolism is affected by the reduction in the process of autophagy. Autophagy and aging are interrelated, and it can be said that increasing age leads to a decrease in autophagy; this decrease can lead to early signs of aging and a short lifespan.

Genetic evidence to highlight the role of autophagy in longevity is present as the loss of macroautophagy reduces the lifespan in worms that carry defective autophagy genes. Moreover, the upregulation of macroautophagy was found in the period of life extension in almost all the experimental models. Similar findings have been reported in flies where there is an increase in age-related diseases with the suppression of autophagy genes.

The defects in the energetic balance of the body as we age are related to a decrease in efficiency of autophagy. Lack of induction of macroautophagy in response to nutritional fluctuations, such as starvation, reduce mobilization of intracellular energy stores and cause loss of protein synthesis through the recycling of amino acids.

Further, a decrease in the autophagy function makes the cells more susceptible to the toxicity of lipid accumulation. The lipid content of cells and tissues is increased with increasing age, and this has a negative effect on the functioning of autophagy. The primary reason behind this is that the lipid content of the cell is crucial for the lipid composition of autophagosomes and related organelles that play a role in the normal function of autophagy. A high level of lipids disrupts the integrity and function of vesicles and lysosomes, thus leading to loss of autophagy in older cells.

HOW WE CAN INDUCE OR PROMOTE AUTOPHAGY

Autophagy is a natural process, but there are specific ways through which it can be induced in the body and one can benefit from the positive effects of autophagy. Some of the most researched and beneficial ways to induce autophagy are given below:

1. Calorie restriction

    - Keto diet

    - Fasting

    - Protein restriction

2. Exercise and high-intensity training

3. Consumption of autophagy-promoting food and supplements

    - Coffee

    - Extra virgin olive oil

    - Turmeric

    - Supplements

5. Quality Sleep

Melany Flores

Calorie Restriction and Autophagy

We are what we eat

Diet has been considered as the most vital factor in governing the health and longevity of humans. Adopting a healthy lifestyle that is comprised of a well-balanced diet and exercise are regarded as the key to good living. In 1935, the concept of calorie restriction (CR) gained remarkable popularity in the field of healthy eating. It was proposed that CR is the most useful dietary intervention that can positively affect longevity and increase lifespan. CR involves a considerable restriction in the intake of calories and lies between the two extremes of food consumption: extremely low food consumption that can lead to starvation and death and extremely high food consumption that can lead to obesity.

There are two main practices of calorie restriction: the keto diet and intermittent fasting. Both these approaches are becoming very popular in health-conscious and/or obese individuals who want to lose weight and become fit. Obesity has become one of the leading causes of a poor lifestyle and a decreased lifespan. The keto diet and intermittent fasting can both play important roles in fighting obesity, and both share a common mechanism of action to improve quality of life, i.e., autophagy.

Mechanism of Anti-Aging Effects of Calorie Restriction

The primary anti-aging effects that result from a controlled diet are due to the role of nutrition in controlling oxidative stress as well as maintaining the genomic and mitochondrial DNA repair mechanism, the concentration of peroxide lipids and protein carbonyls in the tissues and membrane fluidity and functionality. As we age, the oxidative stress in the body is increased while the DNA repair mechanism becomes less efficient and the membrane of the cell loses its fluidity and functionality. However, autophagy is the process that can significantly reduce and reverse these effects of aging as it can influence all these processes.

Selecting the right diet and keeping a check on what we eat is a very critical factor in achieving a long and healthy life. Interestingly, all the signs of aging described above can be regulated by autophagy and related pathways. For instance, calorie restriction has a direct role in suppressing the target of rapamycin (mTOR) which leads to the promotion of autophagy and provides protection against bone disease, motor dysfunction, immune disorders, and insulin sensitivity. CR also decreases the production of IGF-1, which is the primary metabolic intervention that provides protection against age-related diseases and extends one's lifespan. When AMPK is activated, it leads to the downregulation of mTOR and subsequent activation of autophagy. The FOXO gene is also activated by the upregulation of genes related to autophagy and DNA repair, and downregulated by genes that control proliferation and growth of the cell.

Moreover, a nutrient-rich and calorie-restricted diet directly mediates anti-aging effects through upregulation of autophagy. Autophagy functions to provide protection against oxidative stress and eliminates damaged cells and aged organelles from the cell. This allows the cell to become free from unnecessary burdens, dysfunctions, and premature cell death. Autophagy removes the signs of aging from the cell and provides structural and metabolic integrity to it. Various studies suggest that calorie restriction is the most potent inducer of autophagy and has a crucial role in the prevention of age-related diseases.

Keto diet and Autophagia

The trick that makes your body eat your own fat and help you age backwards

What is the keto diet?

The intake of a high-fat diet that is comprised of polyunsaturated fatty acids is termed as the keto diet. The keto diet has a very low intake of carbohydrates, with a fat to carbohydrate ratio of around 5:1.

How does it work?

The keto diet mimics the natural effect of starvation in the body. Ketosis is a natural process that occurs in the human body during lactation and fasting. During ketosis, the body utilizes fats as the primary source of energy instead of carbohydrates through incomplete oxidation of fatty acids. This process occurs in the liver and leads to an increase in the level of acetoacetate and hydroxybutyrate in the body - these are the end products of ketosis.

How ketosis and autophagy are linked?

As the keto diet induces the effects of starvation in the body, it also leads to the induction of autophagy.

Benefits of the Keto Diet

The keto diet has been linked to various health benefits other than the combating of obesity. It has significant neuroprotective effects as this diet leads to an increase in the activity of hypoxia-inducible factor-1α (HIF-1α) and decreased activity of mTORC1 in the hippocampus that leads to the induction of macroautophagy in neurons. Neuronal autophagy has preventive effects on the nervous system against neurodegenerative disorders. Autophagy also leads to the removal of damaged mitochondria that may cause oxidative stress by producing superoxides. It can also remove other protein aggregates that can deteriorate the health of the brain and nervous system. Therefore, through the process of autophagy, the keto diet helps to protect the body against serious conditions like Parkinson's disease, Alzheimer's disease and epilepsy .

Other benefits of a keto diet on the body include:

- Protection against various metabolic syndromes, prediabetes and type 2 diabetes through the loss of fat. It also helps in improving insulin sensitivity.

- Provides protective effects against various heart diseases and ensures the vascular health of an individual.

- Provides protection against cancer, which is attributed to the anti-cancer effects of autophagy.

- Induces autophagy that greatly improves the immune system and helps the body to cope with injuries and diseases in a much better way.

- Improve conditions like polycystic ovary syndrome and acne as both are related to high insulin levels and intake of sugar.

However, for most people it might not be easy to stick to a ketogenic diet for long periods of time, which is why it is essential to find alternative strategies to gain the neuroprotective and other beneficial effects of the keto diet.

Such strategies may include ingestion of coconut oil or other medium-chain triglycerides, intermittent fasting, and the use of supplements that promote ketogenesis, such as carnitine, along with dietary routines that include fasting and cutting down on the intake of carbohydrates. These alternative approaches to promote autophagy in the body are discussed in the next section.

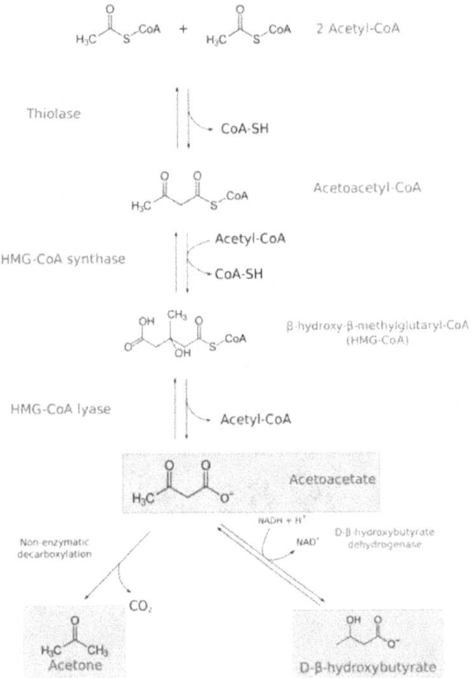

Figure 3. Ketogenesis

Fasting

Fasting is characterized by complete or partial restriction of solid food or water or both for a definite time period. Based on the duration, fasting can be of two types:

- Intermittent fasting (IF) that is characterized by alternate-day fasting of around ≥16 hours or 48 hours of fasting per week.

- Periodic fasting (PF) that is characterized by a minimum of 3 days of fasting in a bi-monthly pattern.

Role of Fasting in Promoting the Anti-Cancer Effects of Autophagy

Fasting has an extraordinary healing effect on the body and has been recognized as one of the most beneficial lifestyle choices that can detox the body and help the rejuvenation of cells and organs. The role of fasting in the induction of autophagy can be considered as a critical feature of the benefits related to fasting. Recently, the role of fasting has shown promising results in promoting anti-cancer effects in the body.

Fasting reduces the ability of tumor cells to use glycolysis as a primary metabolic pathway for the breakdown of glucose and gain energy via a process known as the Warburg effect. Fasting helps in inducing oxidative phosphorylation in tumor cells that lead to increased oxidative stress and reduced levels of lactate and ATP in the cancer cell. As the ADP/ATP ratio is increased, it leads to the activation of the AMPK pathway, which promotes autophagy. Cell death occurs due to a constantly stressful environment. Fasting downregulates the MPAK pathway and suppresses the activation of AKT and mTOR pathways which induce autophagy that leads to the tumor cells' death. Furthermore, fasting also reduces chemotherapy-related damage to the DNA and helps in the early recovery of cells and organs.

Intermittent Fasting and Autophagy

It is not only important that we watch what we eat but also, when we eat.

<u>What is Intermittent Fasting?</u>

The physiology of the human body is quite interesting as it has its own biological clock according to which various processes occur daily. There is a 24-hour light/dark cycle which is controlled by natural circadian oscillators. These circadian oscillators are generally termed as a biological clock and have been conserved throughout the course of evolution. In this way, our body has its own time for various activities, such as being active, resting and regulating our intake of nutrients to ensure optimum function and longevity.

The idea of time-restricted feeding (tRF) has gained considerable attention in the past few years. Various studies in mice have shown that mice that undergo tRF consume the same number of calories in a high-fat diet as compared to the controls, but showed a decreased potential to develop obesity, hepatic steatosis, hyperinsulinemia, and inflammation. The physiological mechanism behind the protective effects of IF includes the regulation of AMPK, mTOR, and CREB pathways. These pathways also improve the cycles of the circadian clock and help in the optimum functioning of our biological clock. Studies suggest that fasting for five days can lead to a 30% decrease in glucose levels in the human body and around 50% decrease in the production of IGF-1, which is an important biomarker of aging and age-related diseases in humans.

Intermittent fasting is one type of time-restricted feeding which involves alternative cycles of eating and fasting. These cycles are comprised of 16 hours of fasting and 8 hours of mealtime, which can include 2 to 3 meals, in 24 hours. There are various types of intermittent fasting, such as the twice a week 16 hours fasting approach, alternate-day fasting, or a complete 24-hour fast once or twice a week. Most of the long-term fasting routines include an extended water fasting regime, which increases the benefits of fasting and promotes autophagy. In each type, intermittent fasting has fantastic benefits on the body.

There are five stages in intermittent fasting that start at 12 hours of fasting and end at 72 hours. Before going into the details of how intermittent fasting affects the body and what happens in each stage, it is necessary to understand what happens in the body when we are not fasting.

In a well-fed cell that has plenty of proteins and carbohydrates, the cell focuses only on dividing and growing. It wastes no time or energy on the cleanup or recycling process. During the growth phase, however, the genes of stress resistance, fat metabolism and damage repair are turned off, and the cell solely focuses on growth.

In the fasting state, the fat in the body is converted into ketone bodies that lead to the reactivation of these genes. These genes lead to the expression of proteins that are involved in the elimination of stress, as body senses starvation as a stress factor. The induced genes function to reduce inflammation, promote DNA repair and cause autophagic degradation of damaged and aged organelles and proteins. In this way, a complete set of proteins and biological processes that lead to the cleansing and replenishing of the cells and tissues are activated.

Fasting induces a self-preservation mode in the cell. It activates AMPK which promotes the breakdown of stored fat and induces autophagy. It also leads to the production of sirtuin proteins that are involved in the synthesis of new mitochondria and reduction of oxidative stress. The formation of ketone bodies during fasting also turn on genes related to damage repair and ant oxidation. All these beneficial processes occur in our body when we don't take in any calories and nutrients, ie., via the time-restricted feeding approach or intermittent fasting.

In the first stage of intermittent and prolonged fasting that is triggered by 12 hours of fasting, the process of ketosis is initiated. In this metabolic process, the body starts using fats as a source of energy. Ketone bodies are formed in the liver and utilized by the brain as an energy source in the absence of glucose. The utilization of ketone bodies by the brain cells help in the removal of inflammation and improve one's mood and mental clarity. By 24 hours of fasting, the cells in the brain and other tissues initiate the process of autophagy to recycle old components and degrade damaged proteins.

Autophagy promotes cellular rejuvenation and frees the cell from the burdens of damaged and inflamed proteins. Autophagy is directly linked with the process of aging, as the presence of inflamed and damaged organelles in the cell is considered as a hallmark of aging. Removal of these signs from the cell by autophagy highlights its importance. In this way, fasting improves the lifespan of an individual.

By 48 hours of low-calorie fasting, the production of various growth hormones is initiated. These hormones play an essential role in cardiovascular protection and in the healing of wounds and injured tissues. Prolonged fasting of 54 to 72 hours initiates the degradation of old immune cells and synthesizes new ones. Autophagy is the primary process that leads to the renewal and revamping of the immune system.

Protein Restriction

Proteins are necessary for the body but only in a limited amount. The importance of a well-balanced diet with respect to protein content is evident from the fact that young individuals who consume a high protein diet where they gain more than 20% of their caloric intake from protein, are more prone to various cancers and have shorter lifespans as compared to individuals who obtain less than 10% of their caloric intake from protein .

The amino acid deficiency during starvation leads to the induction of autophagy as autophagy is regulated by the perfect balance between fuel signaling pathways, mTOR and AMPK. These pathways can be considered as the yin and yang of the human metabolism. mTOR is the primary pathway that regulates the growth and induced anabolism and synthesis of protein. It is activated by the presence of amino acids, glucose and insulin, which leads to the inhibition of autophagy. In contrast to mTOR, the AMPK (AMP-Activated Protein Kinase) is a sensor of catabolism that promotes processes such as oxidation of fat and ketogenesis, and leads to the activation of autophagy. AMPK is activated under energy-deprived conditions, protein restriction, exercise, and fasting.

ROLE OF VARIOUS DIETARY COMPONENTS IN AUTOPHAGY

As we already know that the availability of nutrients regulates the process of autophagy, there are certain dietary components that can directly regulate the level of autophagy. The major macronutrients, including fats, proteins and carbohydrates can mediate the autophagic rate and efficiency in the body. The building blocks of proteins and amino acids are one of the major regulators of autophagy. The presence of amino acids leads to the downregulation or inhibition of autophagy, while the absence of amino acids during the starvation phase leads to the induction of autophagy. Among the different amino acids, the most efficient mediators of autophagy include phenylalanine, leucine and tyrosine. The mTOR pathway mediates the amino acid-based suppression of autophagy as amino acids can increase the intracellular levels of calcium which lead to the activation of the mTOR Complex 1. This complex, when activated, acts as a suppressor of autophagy. The levels of amino acids change according to our diet and intake of proper protein can help regulate the level of autophagy in the cells and body.

Lipids and carbohydrates play an indirect role in the regulation of autophagy. The primary effector of carbohydrates is insulin and levels of this hormone directly mediate the process of autophagy. The catabolism of carbohydrates leads to the release of glucose which is the primary energy source of the cells. Glucose plays an important role in the regulation of endocrine pathways including the insulin pathway. Increased cellular levels of glucose and insulin lead to the activation of the mTOR pathway, which means autophagy is inhibited. Also, the increase in glucose leads to increased levels of NADH through glycolysis which suppresses the activity of sirtuin, another regulator of autophagy. The decreased activity of sirtuin leads to the suppression of autophagy. The presence of high levels of glucose in the cell means that the cell is well fed and the nutrient recycling process, ie., autophagy, is rendered inactive.

The role of fats in the induction of autophagy is quite interesting as high levels of fatty acids in serum develop insulin resistance in the cell. This leads to the inactivation of mTOR which encourages the cell to activate autophagy.

Anti-aging Pharmacological Mimetics for Inducing Autophagy

The challenge of adhering to prolonged CR regimes has led to the development of much safer and convenient alternatives to calorie restriction to achieve autophagy and its anti-aging benefits. Also, there are certain side effects of practicing prolonged CR, which include a delay in healing of wounds and a decrease in body temperature. The search for a pharmacological answer to this has led to the use of various calorie restriction mimetic (CRM) supplements to delay the aging process primarily by the induction of autophagy. The most widely studied and used CRM supplements are spermidine, resveratrol, rapamycin and metformin.

Spermidine

Spermidine is a polyamine that is naturally produced by the body. It is known to play an important role in the determination of lifespan by inducing autophagy. As we age, there is a gradual decline in the production of spermidine. It has been reported that in humans, the use of spermidine dietary supplementation for two months leads to an increase in the blood polyamine concentrations. Spermidine is a non-toxic compound and its use for humans is completely safe. The autophagy-inducing potential of spermidine has been found to be equivalent to rapamycin.

Studies show that the loss of autophagic activity due to the suppression of Atg7 leads to a decrease in lifespan and loss of neuroprotection *in vivo*. In recent decades, the use of spermidine-based dietary supplements has shown promising results in preventing aging and has reduced the risk of Alzheimer's disease. There is experimental evidence that the use of nutritional spermidine leads to delay in age-related memory loss. However, the exact dose for enabling healthy aging by inducing optimal autophagy using spermidine supplements in humans remains unknown.

Resveratrol

Resveratrol is a polyphenol compound. It is naturally obtained from red grapes and blueberry peels. The dietary intake of polyphenols from fruits has gained interest as a preferable source of autophagy induction through calorie restriction effects. Resveratrol is considered as the most potent polyphenol compound. The use of resveratrol has shown positive effects in the treatment and prevention of neurodegenerative diseases. It has been proved to be beneficial for improving age-related cognitive disabilities and has implications in extending the lifespan in yeast models.

There are various physiological effects of resveratrol in the body which mediate its anti-aging and neuroprotective action. Resveratrol causes an increase in the insulin sensitivity, a reduction in IGF1 levels, and activates the AMPK/PGC-1α signaling pathway. It also plays an important role in improving the motor functions of the nervous system. Resveratrol causes a reduction in the inflammatory response caused by the intake of a fat-rich diet and prevents the diet-induced inflammation of the arterial wall.

Despite of having so many benefits for the human body, naturally-occurring resveratrol is poorly absorbed and metabolized by the humans. Hence, various highly effective resveratrol-mimetic drugs, have been developed, for instance, ResVida™. It has been found that the use of resveratrol supplements for one month can lead to a decrease in the levels of circulating glucose, triglycerides, inflammatory markers, and systolic blood pressure. The long-term use of resveratrol supplements has been considered safe for humans.

Longevinex® is another resveratrol supplement that is used commercially. It can induce SIRT1 and has been linked with an increase in levels of Beclin1, LC3-II and FOXO transcription factors. These effects suggest that Longevinex® has beneficial effects on the brain as it increases the rate of mitochondrial biogenesis in the brain and induces neuronal autophagy. Resveratrol can induce the AMPK pathway in the brain cells and can rid the cells from the accumulation of extracellular Aβ by inducing autophagy. Various studies in mice have shown that long term use of resveratrol led to improved memory and reduced the level of Aβ in the brain tissues, which makes it a promising candidate for the treatment of Alzheimer's disease.

Rapamycin

Rapamycin is one of the most widely studied and used autophagy inducers. It is a major suppressor of mTORC1 activity which has been associated to have significant benefits for both health and lifespan in various organisms. It is also one of the most widely used supplements for calorie restriction mimetics. Rapamycin is FDA-approved and can be used for various clinical applications in humans.

Various studies on neurodegenerative disorders using mouse models show that the treatment of affected cells with rapamycin led to an improvement in cognitive ability and reduction in $A\beta$ aggregates. The underlying mechanism of action has been found to be the induction of autophagy, which functions to degrade and remove the aggregates and clears the signs of aging and disease from brain cells. Prolonged use of rapamycin has been found to be associated with expansion of lifespan in mice.

Rapatar is a commercially available formulation of rapamycin. It has a significantly higher bioavailability as compared to naturally-occurring rapamycin. Rapatar has been proven to be beneficial in increasing the lifespan and delaying tumor progression upon lifelong treatment in mice.

Metformin

Metformin is a known drug that is used for the treatment of diabetes. It regulates the blood glucose and insulin levels by targeting various pathways, including the AMPK pathway, mTORC1, insulin/IGF1 pathway, and SIRT1. The regulation of these pathways, which regulate the process of autophagy, makes metformin an important candidate for regulating autophagy in the body. Some of the major metabolic effects of metformin that links its association with autophagy include neuroprotective effects as it lowers the risk of AD in diabetic patients by inducing neuronal autophagy and the removal of Aβ oligomers from brain tissue.

Food that Promotes Autophagy

As autophagy is primarily regulated by the nutrient status of the body, various nutrients and dietary components play an important in the upregulation of autophagy.

Our diet and nutrient intake play an essential role in our body and have far more complex impacts on our body than simply providing energy. The intake of the right nutrients and using food as medicine can have extraordinary effects on our body and its metabolism. Autophagy is a natural process, yet certain foods and nutrients can help in triggering autophagy in our body. Some of these autophagy-promoting foods are given below:

- Consumption of dark-green, leafy vegetables, including kale, spinach, etc., can help in the induction of autophagy in the body. These vegetables are rich in sulforaphane that promote autophagy through the activation of extracellular signal-regulated kinase (ERK) in the nerve cell. Similarly, polyphenols that are also present in green, leafy vegetables and cherries help in promoting autophagy.

- Certain mushrooms, such as the chaga mushroom and various other species are helpful in inducing autophagy in the body.

- Consumption of ginger is advised for the triggering of autophagy as it contains a compound known as 6-shogaol, which induces autophagy through the inhibition of AKT/mTOR pathway in the cells. Turmeric, which contains curcumin, can also induce autophagy through the activation of the AMPK pathway.

- Consuming a considerable amount of coffee is recommended for the induction of autophagy and is part of various diets that are designed to promote autophagy, such as the keto diet. Coffee promotes ketosis, regulates blood sugar, and has a high content of polyphenol, which makes it a perfect triggering factor for autophagy.

- Green tea can trigger autophagy as it is rich in polyphenols. It causes induction of autophagy, especially in liver cells.

- Certain fruits, such as berries, cherries and dark grapes, are recommended to induce autophagy in the body. These fruits contain resveratrol that promotes autophagy.

- Consumption of olive oil (extra virgin) is highly recommended for the induction of autophagy. It contains various polyphenols such as oleuropein and oleocanthal, which trigger autophagy through the suppression of mTOR.

- Various foods such as salmon, algae, mackerel and flax seeds are also considered as important sources of autophagy inducers. These contain omega-3 polyunsaturated fatty acids that induce autophagy.

- Similarly, eggs, liver, pumpkin seeds and red meat are also beneficial in the triggering of autophagy. The presence of a high amount of zinc acts as an essential inducer of autophagy in the body.

Autophagy-Inducing Foods

There are certain foods and food components that are widely researched for therapeutic purposes due to their autophagy-inducing abilities. These dietary components provide a natural means for the treatment of various diseases, including neurodegenerative diseases, metabolic disorders, and cancers. The mechanism of action of these foods is primarily the induction of autophagy. However, there are various direct and indirect cellular pathways of autophagy that are influenced by the active components of the food. Some of the most widely studied and most effective food and food components that can lead to the induction of autophagy in the cells are given below:

Caffeine

Caffeine is the major active component of cocoa, tea and coffee. It is also added to colas and drinks as a flavoring agent. Caffeine can induce autophagy in the body. Various studies suggest that treatment of microbial cells with a small concentration of caffeine can lead to induction of autophagy. In humans, caffeine acts an inducer of autophagy as it inhibits the production of various kinase enzymes that are part of mTOR pathway. Caffeine also plays various roles in other vital processes of the cells, including apoptosis, and affects cell cycle regulatory proteins such as p53. Caffeine also has positive effects on the health of our brain and neurological system. It can improve our cognitive abilities and has been shown to help patients with neurodegenerative diseases, such as Parkinson's, in managing their symptoms. It is assumed that these neuroprotective effects of caffeine are attributed to the induction of autophagy in brain cells. Consumption of coffee and other caffeine-containing products have been linked with an increase in lifespan, a trait that is also attributed to autophagy.

Curcumin

Curcumin is a natural compound that is present in turmeric. It is the active component of turmeric which gives the yellow color to curry and has a distinct taste. Curcumin is a biologically active compound and has been used in various therapeutic medicines, including anticancer drugs. The mechanism of action of curcumin involves its vital role in the production of the autophagosome, and thereby, autophagy. It induces cell death in abnormal cells through the activation of autophagy. Treatment of various cancerous cell lines with a controlled amount of curcumin has been shown to cause an increase in the production of autophagic vesicles and autophagosomes in cells. This increase leads to the destruction and death of the cancerous cells and thus depicts the anti-cancer potential of turmeric. A daily dose of up to 100 mg/day can be ingested from food and is considered nontoxic. The bioavailability of ingested curcumin is quite low but can be enhanced by ingesting pepper with curcumin, which contains piperine. Curcumin has been a part of traditional medicine since early times. The use of turmeric has been beneficial for curing various inflammatory and neurodegenerative diseases, primarily due to its autophagic potential.

Fenugreek

Fenugreek is a leguminous plant, native to countries in Asia and the Middle East. It is used in various forms, including whole-seed and ground-state as a source of protein. The active component of fenugreek has been shown to induce vacuolization in various tissues which suggests its autophagic role. Various studies suggest that fenugreek extracts have protective effects against cancer as cells exposed to cancer-inducing compounds failed to affect the fenugreek-treated cells as compared to untreated cells. The treated cells showed an increased amount of autophagosomes that contained damaged organelles and other cytoplasmic materials and hence protected the cell through autophagy.

Vitamin C

Vitamin C is found in many vegetables and fruits and is most prevalent in citrus fruits. It is also known as ascorbic acid and it provides amazing health benefits. Vitamin C has anti-cancer properties and studies suggest that the treatment of cancer cells with vitamin C induces the production of autophagic vesicles and leads to the removal of damaged organelles and cells. Similarly, patients with neurodegenerative diseases have a low level of vitamin C in the serum, which suggests a low level of autophagy that can cause problems with the neuronal system and neurodegeneration. A daily intake of around five fruits and vegetables is equivalent to 250 mg of vitamin C, which is enough to meet the bioavailability of vitamin C in the body and meet our body's needs.

Vitamin D

One of the most important and prevalent components of our diet is calcium and vitamin D. Various analogs and supplements of calcium and vitamin D are used along with natural sources such as fish, dairy products and the sun to fulfill the nutrient requirements of our body. The effect of vitamin D on various human tissues shows that there was an increase in the production of autophagosomes and the process of autophagy. Vitamin D mediates the levels of calcium in the body, which influences the mTOR pathway. The inhibition of mTOR leads to the induction of the autophagic process. Various studies show the protective role of vitamin D against breast, ovarian and colon cancer. The primary mechanism of action through which vitamin D confers anti-cancer effects is through autophagic destruction and death of cancerous cells.

Sulphoraphane

Sulphoraphane is a potent anti-cancer compound found in various plants, including cruciferous vegetables. This compound affects various vital processes in the cell, including the cell cycle, apoptosis, protection from genotoxic damage and autophagy. Sulphoraphane has shown positive effects on cancerous cells from prostate tissues, where treatment with this compound led to an increase in the autophagic structures in the cells. The cytoprotective effects of autophagy were found to be associated with a decline in the release of cytochrome, which helps in the destruction of cancerous cells. Sulphoraphane also affects the expression of Bcl-2; decrease in Bcl-2 leads to the activation of Beclin-1. And as described above, Beclin-1 plays an important role in the activation of autophagy.

Tocotrienols

These compounds are derivates of vitamin E and are naturally present in rice bran and palm oil. They have neuroprotective and anti-tumor properties and various studies suggest that these health-promoting effects of tocotrienols are attributed to their ability to induce autophagy in the cells.

Lithium

Lithium belongs to a group of alkali metals in the periodic table. It is naturally present in meat, grains, vegetables, and water. Animal studies show that the treatment of kidney cells with lithium causes an increase in the number of autophagosomes. This autophagic effect was elicited through the inhibition of inositol monophosphate rather than the mTOR signaling pathway. The autophagy-inducing ability of lithium has been linked with its role in protection against Huntington disease, which is a neurodegenerative disorder that is characterized by the formation and accumulation of huntingtin protein aggregates in the body. Moreover, the role of lithium in the induction of autophagy can be exploited for the degradation and removal of mutant α-synuclein protein aggregates, which cause Parkinson's disease.

Luteolin

Luteolin is a naturally occurring flavone. It is found in celery, chamomile tea, green pepper and perilla seeds. It has been identified as a down regulator of the autophagic process. Luteolin has anti-tumorigenic properties and has shown positive results in the treatment of oral squamous cell carcinoma. Luteolin inhibits autophagy, which helps the survival and progression of cancer cells as they avoid apoptosis. Therefore, by reducing autophagy, we can induce apoptosis or cell death of cancer cells which can aid in anti-cancer therapy.

MK615

MK615 is a natural compound. It is obtained from Japanese apricot and has anticancer properties. MK615 can inhibit the proliferation of breast cancer cells and induce apoptosis in them, leading to cell death. Furthermore, upon treatment with MK615, there was an increase in the number of autophagic vesicles in the cancerous cells. Similar findings have been reported from studies on colon cancer cells which highlight the ant proliferative and apoptosis-inducing effects of MK615, which are attributed to autophagy.

Apigenin

A major regulator of autophagy that is found in a wide range of herbs and plants is apigenin. It is present in pepper, oregano, thyme, parsley, rosemary, olives, and celery.

Benzyl Isothiocyanate

Benzyl isothiocyanate is primarily present in cruciferous vegetables. It has been known to have chemoprotective properties. Treatment of breast cancer cells with a controlled amount of benzyl isothiocyanate led to cell cycle arrest, apoptosis, and an increase in the production of autophagosomes.

Bromovanin

Bromovanin is present in vanillin and gives the distinct flavor and aroma of vanilla. Various studies suggest that the treatment of various cells with bromovanin led to an increase in the production of the autophagosome, thus marking the induction of autophagy. Bromovanin can also induce apoptosis, decrease the activity of certain kinases, and increase the production of ROS (reactive oxygen species), which also promote autophagy.

Triterpenoid Saponins (Group B)

These compounds are present primarily in soya products and are termed as soyasaponins. They are a subclass of triterpenoids which have various health benefits. Triterpenoids are predominant in intact legumes and have been investigated for their effects on autophagy. Soy products contain B-group triterpenoids, which includes saponins and genistein. They have anti-cancer properties. High amount of soy products in the diet have been linked with decreased levels of prostate and breast cancer, and these anti-cancer effects have been linked to an increase in the production of autophagic vesicles upon treatment with saponins and genistein.

Autophagy and Weight Loss

The importance of autophagy and autophagy-inducing factors in controlling the weight of the body has been highlighted in recent years. Autophagy is a catabolic process that influences the nutrient status of the body. Furthermore, it also mediates the process of fat metabolism and glucose levels in the body. Various studies in mice models show that induction of autophagy through calorie restriction led to weight loss in healthy mice as compared to the experimental mice which lack the autophagy gene *atg4b*. These findings suggest that there is a definitive role of autophagy in controlling body mass and weight. The systemic activity of autophagy provides protection forth organism against gain weight when subjected to a diet that is rich in calories.

Exercise, Training, and Autophagy

Physical activity increases strength, endurance and makes our metabolism top notch

The Difference between Exercise and Training

Exercise and training refers to both physical activity and workouts. However, there is a certain technical difference between the two as exercise is performed to get immediate effects from a workout, such as burning calories, building biceps, stretching, and shedding some sweat, whereas training is a physical activity that is designed and performed to achieve a goal and is about the process of learning something through specific physical exercise and endurance activities.

In both forms, physical activity is considered as an important factor for the health and wellbeing of the body. And one of the most vital roles of exercise in the body is that it acts as a trigger for autophagy.

Benefits of Exercise In Relation to Autophagy

Exercise causes a sharp increase in the consumption of oxygen and energy that results in the decrease of nutrients and oxygen, and an increase in oxidative stress by the generation of reactive oxygen species (ROS). These cellular conditions act as a trigger for the process of autophagy that aids the cell in coping with a stressful environment.

Exercise-induced autophagy has been observed in various tissues and organs of the body. For instance, the liver, adipose tissues, skeletal muscle, pancreas, cardiac muscle, and cerebral cortex are some of the most significant issues that undergo exercise-induced autophagy. Physical exercise has many beneficial effects on our health, which includes an increase the in life-span, and protects the body from diabetes, neurodegenerative disorders and various types of cancers — most of the health benefits of exercise overlap with known protective roles of autophagy.

Various studies suggest that exercise and training can increase the rate of autophagy to maintain the physiological activities of skeletal muscle. Other benefits of exercise that primarily affect the health of cardiac tissues involve the inhibition of apoptosis that has occurred due to myocardial infarction, reduction in myocardial cell damage and improvement of cardiovascular function. Aerobic exercise induces autophagy that protects cardiac cells.

Proper exercise and training at a favorable intensity can induce autophagy that helps in the degradation and removal of metabolic waste that is necessary to maintain the steady-state of the cell.

Improving Energy Metabolism

Exercise and training play an important role in enhancing the metabolic system and efficiency in the body. It does so by affecting the turnover rate of mitochondria. This means that it improves the synthesis of mitochondria and induces autophagy to remove the aged or damaged mitochondria from the cell. In this way, exercise ensures that enough healthy mitochondria that function at their best and maintain the proficiency of metabolism are present. Moreover, autophagy and microRNA-mediated autophagy are involved in the regulation of the removal of unwanted organelles from the cell and promote the adaptation of muscles and metabolism towards exercise.

Various studies have researched the role of exercise in the induction of autophagy in multiple tissues and parts of the body. Some of the most significant tissues where exercise-related autophagy is triggered are skeletal muscles which are discussed below.

Autophagy in Skeletal Muscles

The role of exercise training in mediating the process of autophagy has become a hot spot in the field of exercise science. In 1984, it was reported that endurance exercise and high-intensity workouts promote the induction of autophagy in skeletal muscle. Experiments on mice that were subjected to high-intensity treadmill training showed that the strongest autophagy response was observed within 48 hours after exercise.

Exercise and training accelerate the metabolic processes involving the catabolism and anabolism of fatty acids, proteins, and, glucose. It also promotes the biogenesis of mitochondria, influences the process of angiogenesis, and causes a delay in the aging of skeletal muscle. All these effects are attributed to the process of autophagy that is induced by exercise training.

High-altitude training leads to the induction of the process of autophagy which eventually improves exercise performance. High-altitude training induces autophagy and mitophagy that aids in the maintenance of the quality of skeletal muscle by eliminating abnormal and aged mitochondria from the cell. This cleansing process promotes the efficiency of energy metabolism that is required by the cell to fulfill the increased energy needs.

High altitude training also leads to the activation of HIF-1 that stimulates the expression of vascular endothelial factor (VEGF) and erythropoietin (EPO). These growth factors increase the mass of hemoglobin and the density of capillaries in the muscle.

Autophagy prepares the body and strengthens the metabolic process of the cell to endure exercise and high-altitude training. Aerobic and hypoxic training exercises lead to the induction of autophagy, which suggests that autophagy is the molecular mechanism of the adaptive response of the body to exercise and high-altitude training. The production of autophagic biomarkers during endurance exercises and high-altitude training might provide useful insight into the potential of an individual for such training. However, extreme exercise and training can cause excessive autophagy that can lead to excessive degradation of protein and loss of skeletal muscle.

Thus, we can say that autophagy in skeletal muscle plays a significant role in maintaining its quality and structure. The regulation of protein degradation as well synthesis of proteins by autophagy is equally vital for ensuring the health of skeletal muscles after endurance exercise and training.

Mechanism of autophagy in Skeletal Muscles

Various changes in the biochemistry of autophagy in the skeletal muscles help the muscles adapt to its changing energy needs. When muscles are subjected to bouts of high-intensity exercise, it leads to the induction of autophagy in both oxidative and glycolytic muscles. It also leads to a reduction in the synthesis of proteins during the exercise period and an increase in protein synthesis later in the recovery period. For young adults, the use of acute-endurance training proves to be more beneficial, while the use of resistance-training in older age can have similar benefits on the body as both induce autophagy and help in improving the strength and endurance of the muscles.

Doing an Autophagy Session

Autophagy can be induced through the right diet and exercise, so it is highly recommended that we treat ourselves with the extraordinary benefits of autophagy. It is a natural detox process for our body and helps us achieve the desirable concept of *healthy aging*!

After reading the above section, we can pick some quick and easy tips that will help in the induction of autophagy in our body:

1. Practice a high-intensity training session that is comprised of sprints and strength training as this will trigger autophagy.

2. To increase autophagy, fasting for two or three days a week is highly recommended.

3. It is very beneficial to stay active and on our feet throughout our fast. This will help ramp up the metabolism of fats and lead to ketosis, which further induces autophagy in our cells.

4. During intermittent fasting, drink as much coffee as possible as it is a strong inducer of autophagy.

5. Follow a high-fat, low-carbohydrate diet plan and limit your protein intake. This diet plan will boost the process of autophagy.

6. Get proper sleep so that your body can rest and recover through autophagy.

Autophagy Inducing Supplements and Therapies

Apart from diet and exercise, there are certain supplements and therapies that are used at the clinical level to induce autophagy. Such clinical approaches have gained worldwide attention as autophagy acts as a natural cleanser of the body and hence has a significant role in the elimination and treatment of various ailments and diseases.

Moreover, multiple supplements and compounds have been developed that artificially induce autophagy in the body. This is a novel approach to autophagy regulation as most of these supplements do not require mTOR for the induction of the autophagic process and can independently regulate it. Some of the few FDA approved compounds that are used for promoting autophagy in humans are given in **Table 4.**

Table 4. The list of compounds that have the potential to induce autophagy

Sr #	Compounds	Autophagy Induction Mechanism
1	Carbamazepine	Decreases the level of inositol in the body
2	Sodium valproate	Decreases the level of inositol in the body
3	Metformin	Decreases the level of AMPK and induces beclin1 and ULK1
4	Verapamil	Decreases the level of intra-cytosolic calcium
5	Clonidine	Decreases the level of cAMP in the cells
6	Tyrosine kinase inhibitors	Induces the level of beclin1 and inhibits mTOR
7	Trifluoperazine	Mechanism not known
8	Rilmenidine	Decreases the level of cAMP in the cells
9	Rapamycin	Inhibits the production of mTORC1
10	Statins	Activates the production of AMPK
11	Lithium	Decreases the level of inositol in the body

There are some nutritional supplements that are recommended by physicians to promote the process of autophagy (**Table 5**).

Table 5. List of dietary supplements that have the potential to induce autophagy

Sr #	Compounds	Autophagy Induction Mechanism
1	Vitamin D	Induces transcriptional genes through calcium signaling
2	Resveratrol	Induces sirtuin 1
3	Caffeine	Suppresses mTOR signaling
4	Spermidine	Inhibits acetylase
5	Trehalose	Not known
6	Omega-3 polyunsaturated fatty acid	Inhibits the signaling of m-TOR

Clinical Approaches to Induce Autophagy

Various clinical approaches are used to regulate and induce autophagy in the body. Three of the most common therapeutic methods related to autophagy are given below:

- Autophagy gene therapy

- Transgenic expression of autophagy

- Autophagy-inducing peptides

The systemic expression of the autophagy-related gene Atg5 has been shown to induce positive effects in mice models. It has led to the expansion of the lifespan, and an end-efficient metabolism profile.

Various autophagy-related genes are being used as targets to improve various clinical conditions. Gene therapy involves the tissue-specific delivery of autophagic genes using different vectors or carriers. Through this method, the most important autophagy-related genes, including Atg7, Beclin-1 and Tfeb have been delivered to liver, brain, and muscle cells to aid in the treatment of various liver and muscular disorders.

Autophagy-related gene therapies have shown an improvement in the function of hepatic insulin and systemic glucose tolerance in mice. They have also shown positive results in the treatment of lysosomal storage muscle disease in muscles, such as Pompe disease. Gene therapy using autophagy-related genes have great potential in treating neurodegenerative diseases, such as Parkinson's and Alzheimer's disease.

Various autophagy-inducing peptides, including Tat-Beclin-1, have been shown to have therapeutic potential as this peptide is designed to induce autophagy in multiple diseased cells and tissues.

Screening for Autophagy-Inducing CRMs

Among various nutritional and chemical supplements that are used to induce autophagy in the body, the use of autophagy-inducing drugs for the attenuation of risks that are associated with different age-associated diseases is becoming common. Recently, an autophagic flux probe has been developed. This probe can analyze and rank different autophagy-inducing drugs based on their potency level by screening through a known drug library. The autophagic flux probe is GFP-LC3-RFP-LC3ΔG. It is a fusion protein and gives out a signal when autophagy occurs in the body; this signal is then analyzed against a candidate drug that is being screened for its autophagy-inducing potential. A low GFP/RFP ratio indicates a strong autophagy inducer. By using this approach, various autophagy inducers have been identified. They are specified in Table 6 along with the pathologies for which the drugs have been proved to be beneficial by inducing autophagy.

Table 6. The list of useful drugs for the induction of autophagy identified via probe method

Serial #	Drug	Disease	GFP/RFP (%)
1	Ciclopirox olamine	Cancer	1
2	Cladribine (2-CDA)	Alzheimer's Disease	51.1
3	Sertraline hydrochloride	Depression	58.8
4	Loperamide hydrochloride	Hematopoiesis disorders	70
5	Azacytidine	Huntington Disease	61.7

Various antiaging nutrients that induce autophagy have been identified using this probe. These nutrients include antioxidants, which include vitamins A, D, and E and related coenzymes, as well as various phytochemicals including curcumin.

The Ideal Diet for Successful Aging

Nutrition transition and preferable dietary patterns have evolved around the world and different regions and cultures have unique eating habits. It has been found that regions including Asia, Middle East, Latin America and sub-Saharan African countries have relatively similar dietary patterns. Various studies on age-associated diseases and dietary patterns have highlighted the role of nutrients and food with the increased risk of age-associated diseases in this region. This region has become bound to the consumption of high fat and high sugar foods, and this commonality is proportional to the ratio of age-associated diseases in the people of these regions.

On the other hand, in regions where the Okinawan diet is common, people are less prone to age-related disorders. This diet includes low-GI grains, sweet potatoes, leguminous plants, carotenoid-rich food and different kinds of flavonoids. Such a dietary regime is considered as part of calorie restriction (CR) practices and has been considered to be the most advantageous dietary choice for successful aging. The underlying process behind the benefits of such a calorie-restricted diet has been found to be autophagy, which cleanses the body and plays an important role in achieving longevity.

Melany Flores

Sleep as a Regulator of Autophagy

Sleep better and recover faster through autophagy

Sleep is considered a necessary and effective treatment of various conditions as it is the time when our body rests and heals itself. The sleep and wake cycle are an essential part of the circadian rhythm, or the internal biological clock of the body. The natural clock of our body regulates all the vital processes in our body. Autophagy is among one of them.

The activation of autophagy in cells is well controlled and follows a rhythmic cycle. The natural biological clock works according to the division of day and night, or a cycle of sleep and wakefulness. Sleep acts as an essential regulator of autophagy and disruption of sleep cycles. A lack of sleep can affect the functionality of the circadian rhythm and can compromise the accuracy and efficiency of autophagy.

There is a close coupling between the biological clock and the autophagic degradation process that maintains energy homeostasis in the body. This coupling also helps in the remodeling of cell organelles and proteins, compartmentalization of tissue metabolism, and provides a balance of nutrients. The circadian autophagy is regulated by two cues, the time of day and nutritional signals. So, if we follow the natural sleep and wakefulness cycle as determined by our biological clock, the process of the circadian rhythm of autophagy also works in an optimum manner to regulate vital metabolic processes.

Getting good quality sleep has been linked with a healthy body and mind whereas sleep deprivation is associated with various neurological and physiological disorders and a decrease in lifespan. The importance of sleep is due to the different essential processes that occur during sleeping, and a lack of sleep causes disruption of these vital physiological processes.

The vital processes that occur during sleep include the physical repair of muscles and organs, muscle growth, consolidation of memory, loss of fat and autophagy. Moreover, sleep is vital for brain functions as various toxic proteins and beta-amyloid are cleared from the brain through autophagy. This autophagic removal of beta-amyloid is crucial in the protection from Alzheimer's disease.

Moreover, autophagy is regulated by certain hormones. Melatonin, that is a sleep hormone that greatly influences autophagy. It prepares the body for beneficial processes such as growth and repair through autophagy. Autophagy also occurs in during the diurnal rhythm in heart, muscles, and liver in mice and has an increased rate at periods of low metabolic activity such as sleep. Furthermore, nearly all metabolic processes including the biosynthesis of cholesterol, beta-oxidation of fatty acids and gluconeogenesis in the liver, occur at rhythmical cycles and autophagy is involved in these processes to ensure nutrient supply for oxidation as well as storage. Thus, autophagy is intensely regulated by the biological clock and our sleep-wakefulness cycles. Ensuring proper and deep sleep helps our body to cleanse and repair itself through autophagy.

The recommended amount of sleep varies from 6 to 8 hours; however, time and quality of sleep are more significant than the number of sleeping hours. A few hours of sound sleep at night is more beneficial than sleeping for long hours during the daytime. Following the sleep cycle as determined by our biological clock and maintaining the circadian rhythms of the body will upregulate the process of autophagy and improve our health and lifespan. A lack of sleep causes the internal clock to become out of sync with the environment and can lead to stress and inflammation in the body.

AUTOPHAGY AND OBESITY

Autophagy is a degradative process. It plays an important role in managing various stresses in the body, including obesity and related stresses. These stresses include oxidative stresses, proteotoxic stress, and obesity-associated toxicity. Obesity is a global problem that affects around 2.1 billion people, approximately 30% of the population. Autophagy helps in maintaining the homeostasis of the body by coping with the stresses related to obesity. However, obesity can compromise or inhibit the process of autophagy at various levels. This can lead to worsening of obesity-related metabolic pathologies that can cause dysfunction in multiple organs.

On the other hand, there are certain studies that suggest that the inhibition of autophagy under certain conditions can have beneficial effects in reducing various damaging consequences of obesity. So, autophagy plays a dual role in obesity and related pathologies. It can protect as well as promote the damages of obesity under different conditions. This role of autophagy highlights its importance in the metabolic and physiological pathways of the body, as obesity is a multifactorial disease and results in pathologies that may affect various organs of the body. For instance, obesity is commonly associated with diverse comorbidities, including cardiovascular disease, hypertension, diabetes, dyslipidemia and cancer. The autophagic catabolism plays a significant role in preventing the complications of obesity and a lack of autophagy can have deleterious effects on the health, especially in obese individuals.

Stresses Related to Obesity

The major cause of obesity is our modern lifestyle, which primarily entails a lack of physical activity, an unhealthy diet, and over-nutrition. This has led to the current epidemic of obesity and it is getting worse with every passing day. Obesity results from the consumption of surplus calories that get stored as fat in the adipose tissue. The accumulation of fat can also occur in non-adipose tissue, including the skeletal muscles and liver, which can be damaging to these tissues. Moreover, the accumulation of excessive fat can increase the level of free fatty acids in the serum which is characterized as systemic lipotoxicity.

All biological membranes have lipids as an integral part of their system. The presence of excessive influx and accumulation of lipids can affect cellular function by altering the fluidity and integrity of their membranes. Obesity can lead to changes in the lipidomic profile of various organelles, including the endoplasmic reticulum (ER). This can compromise the process of protein synthesis and lead to the accumulation of unfolded proteins. These unfolded proteins have toxic effects on the ER which leads to lipogenesis. The proteotoxic effects can also trigger various lipotoxic pathologies. Presence of high level of lipids can induce various stress responses, including oxidative stress by the production of ROS, the stress of signaling pathway, and stress-activated protein kinase signaling that triggers obesity-related metabolic pathologies. The metabolites of fatty acids can indirectly activate stress signaling pathways in the cell. Together, these responses lead to a magnification of pathologies or complications of obesity, such as insulin resistance and chronic inflammation.

Autophagy is a major stress-combating process of the body and helps the cells in maintaining their function by fighting off various stresses. Autophagy plays a protective role against the lipid-induced stresses in the following ways:

- Autophagy eliminates and destroys the lipid droplets through the process called lipophagy. This reduces the fat content and normalizes the metabolism of lipids in the tissues of obese individuals.

- Autophagy eliminates dysfunctional mitochondria through a process called mitophagy. This reduces the production of ROS and protects the cells from obesity-associated pathologies and DNA damage.

- During ER stress, autophagy can fight ER stress by eliminating a part of the ER through a process called ER-phagy. This removes the damaged parts of the ER and restores its homeostasis.

In this way, autophagy plays a very crucial role in the resolution of obesity-associated stresses in the body and provides protection against the clinical complications of obesity. However, it has been reported that obesity and obesity-related stresses can interfere with the process of autophagy and make it ineffective. The absence of autophagy in the cells can make them vulnerable to the damages of obesity. There are various ways through which obesity and related stresses can compromise autophagic process. They will be discussed in the next section.

Effects of Obesity on Autophagy

Initially, it was believed that the process of autophagy is inactive during obesity. In conditions of hyper-nutrition when the cell is well fed, the autophagy process is turned off by the inhibition of AMPK and activation of mTORC1. Various studies suggest that the activity of mTORC1 is triggered during obesity and is linked with an increase in the synthesis of energy reserves in the liver. Many studies that involved obese mice show that there is a downregulation of the autophagic process in test subjects. Genetic analysis shows a reduction in expression of the ATG5 and ATG7 genes that indicate a decrease in the production of the autophagosome. The comorbidities of obesity, insulin resistance and hyper-insulinemia also have inhibitory effects on the process of autophagy during obesity. The lipotoxic stress can decrease the AMPK signaling which can decrease the production of the autophagosome in various cells, including liver cells and macrophages.

All these studies suggest that the process of autophagy is downregulated by obesity and its related stresses. However, recent studies in human and mouse tissues show that there is an increase in the production of autophagosomes in response to obesity and related lipotoxic stress in various tissues, including adipose and liver tissues. These findings show that the connection between autophagy and obesity is not as simple as was speculated originally, and that autophagy plays a more crucial role in obesity and related pathologies.

There is more evidence that autophagy process is upregulated in obesity. It has been reported that ER stress—the hallmark of obesity and lipotoxicity— can cause the induction of autophagy via several mechanisms. Obesity itself is a strong inducer of ER stress in the liver cells. Obesity-associated ER stress increases the accumulation of fat in various tissues and cause insulin resistance and damage to liver cells. In this way, autophagy is induced by obesity and related stresses as a defensive mechanism to protect cells from the damages of ER stress.

In fibroblasts, protein kinase C (PKC) is activated by the lipotoxic effects on the cell. The activation of this protein upregulates the autophagic flux which protects the cell from apoptosis. Other stresses linked to obesity include oxidative stress and inflammation and have also been reported as strong inducers of autophagy. These stresses can upregulate autophagy via multiple pathways. In obesity-related stress, the induction of autophagy can be characterized as a cellular defense mechanism. It ensures cell survival by maintaining the cellular homeostasis in unfavorable stress conditions.

However, the induction of autophagy in lipid-overloaded cells should result in a decrease in the accumulation of lipid droplets. However, the findings show the opposite reaction. The autophagic process fails to decrease this accumulation and there is an increase in substrate levels in various cells due to obesity and lipotoxicity. These findings propose that obesity can interfere with the efficiency of autophagy.

Studies have shown that there is an increase in the production of autophagosomes in cells of obese individuals, but the actual parameter that determines the efficiency of autophagy process, the autophagic flux, is reduced. So, the upregulation of autophagy as evident by the production of vesicles can be seen in obesity and associated stresses, but the process is not carried out in the way it should be. There is a certain kind of interference from the obesity-associated stresses that lead to a fizzled autophagic process.

This defect in the degradative abilities of autophagy is of the leading causes of the accumulation of autophagosomes during obesity. Such accumulation has been reported in pancreatic beta cells, as well as liver and kidney cells from obese individuals. The inhibition of catabolic action of autophagy in obese individuals is carried out by various mechanisms.

It has been reported that lipotoxic stress can interfere with the autophagic flux through different mechanisms in different tissues. Thus, this inhibition of autophagic flux is a tissue-dependent mechanism and varies according to the tissues in which autophagy have been induced under obesity-related stresses.

For instance, in the liver cells, the process of autophagy was stalled at the step of autophagosome-lysosome fusion. The primary reason behind this failure was found to be the increased level of calcium in the cell due to lipotoxicity. The increased lipids in the cell membrane compromise the action of calcium channels in the membrane, leading to dysregulation in autophagy. This mechanism of autophagic flux inhibition is termed calcium-dependent mechanism of inhibition.

Lipotoxicity and obesity can induce the expression of a special inhibitory protein called Rubicon. This protein functions to inhibit the fusion between autophagosomes and lysosome in a calcium-independent mechanism of autophagic flux inhibition.

The cells of the kidney do not show errors in the step of autophagosome-lysosome fusion under obesity-related stresses. They display another mechanism of inhibition of autophagic flux and display a defect in the lysosomal acidification. The optimum pH of the lysosome is essential for its normal functions and degradative abilities. The increased acidification of lysosomal enzymes can lead to impairment of the cargo degradation process, which is the essence of autophagy. Lipotoxicity can impair the degradative or catabolic abilities of autophagy and thus decrease the autophagic flux in kidney cells.

In pancreatic beta cells, both types of defects in the autophagy processes have been observed under obesity stresses. The failure of autophagosome-lysosome fusion and acidification of lysosomes were both detected after lipotoxic insults. Thus, the autophagy inhibitory mechanisms of lipotoxicity that decrease the autophagic flux vary with tissues and cell types.

Role of Autophagy in Obesity-Related Pathologies

The complex and intricate relationship between the process of autophagy and obesity suggest that autophagy plays a critical role in the regulation of the different pathologies related to obesity. As we know, obesity can have various complications and pathologies which can lead to increased lipid content in cells, accumulation of aggregates of damaged proteins and can cause harm to mitochondrial function. All the pathological effects of autophagy are also a primary substrate of the autophagic process. In this way, autophagy can govern the extent of pathological effects of obesity on the body and can determine the level of complications caused by obesity-related stresses in the body. And the failure or termination of the autophagic process can lead to acceleration in the obesity-associated pathologies in several organs.

Genetic studies have shown that the loss of autophagy genes in liver cells tend to have similar phenotypic effects as observed in obesity-associated non-alcoholic steatohepatitis (NASH). These pathological indications include the formation of protein inclusion bodies, accumulation of fat and liver injury. These findings suggest that obesity and autophagy are strongly interrelated, and that pathologies related to obesity can worsen in cells with defective autophagic machinery. It has been reported that the systemic reduction in the activity of the autophagic process due to the Atg7 gene insufficiency can accelerate the progression of diabetic pathologies in obese individuals. So, the presence of genetic defects in the autophagic system in obese individuals is related to high rates of morbidity and mortality.

However, the over expression of the Atg5 gene, which functions to increase the process of autophagy, has a protective effect on mice against age-associated obesity and insulin resistance. The over expression of Atg7 gene in liver cells showed an improvement in the obesity-associated ER stress. These findings confirm the protective role of autophagy in the body against obesity-related pathologies.

Various therapeutic approaches have been developed to manipulate the process of autophagy to gain benefits for obesity-related pathologies and stresses. For instance, autophagy flux is increased in liver cells by treatment with autophagy-inducing compounds such as carbamazepine and rapamycin. These compounds induce autophagy and help in the catabolic removal of accumulated fats from the liver cells and aid in the healing of injury to the liver. Various calcium blockers are used to restore the autophagic flux in liver cells of obese individuals. These compounds also showed promising results in normalizing the levels of fats and insulin resistance in cases of obesity caused by the consumption of a high-fat diet.

The genetic removal of Rubicon can lead to the restoration of autophagosome-lysosome fusion during obesity-related lipotoxic effects. This restoration of the autophagic process leads to the catabolic removal of accumulated fats from the cell and rids the cell of the toxic effects of obesity. These findings suggest that autophagy provides protection against obesity-related pathologies in liver cells.

However, there are certain studies that suggest the opposite role of autophagy in the determination of obesity-related pathologies in the body. Knockout studies of the Atg7 gene in mice liver and skeletal muscle cells resulted in positive effects on various pathologies related to obesity. These include insulin resistance, adipogenesis, and accumulation of fat. The reason behind these effects upon termination of autophagy is attributed to the synthesis of a special metabolic protein, FGF21, that carries out the metabolism of accumulated lipids in a tissue-specific manner. In similar findings, mice with deletion of the FIP200 gene that is essential for the formation of autophagosomes in the liver cells showed decreased levels of hepatic injury in obese individuals.

These findings suggest a very interesting role of autophagy in the homeostasis of the body and especially in pathologies related to obesity. They show that the process of autophagy plays an important role in controlling the pathological stresses of obesity, but in certain conditions, these stresses overcome the efficiency of autophagy and make it more harmful rather than beneficial for the cell. On the other hand, the complete termination of the autophagic process due to lipotoxic stress can lead to the induction of other compensatory mechanisms that cannot be compromised by the obesity-associated stresses. This process can successfully protect the cells from the complication of obesity and autophagy malfunction. So, in certain cells types, there is a failsafe mechanism that operates in the cell when the process of autophagy has been compromised by the lipotoxic and other stresses induced by obesity.

Autophagy plays an important role in the modification of the pathological outcome of obesity in the macrophages of hepatic stellate cells. The absence of autophagy in these macrophages can lead to an increase in inflammation. Autophagy plays an important role in maintaining the health of the vascular system and inhibition of autophagy due to obesity can lead to a major cardiovascular pathology known as atherosclerosis. Autophagy mediates the process of inflammation in the immune cells and functions to reduce obesity-associated inflammation and other pathologies.

On the other hand, the inhibition of autophagy in hepatic stellate cells leads to a decrease in fibrosis and injury of liver tissue. The inhibition of autophagy in beta cells leads to loss of function and triggers various diabetes-related symptoms, including increased blood sugar level and glucose intolerance, as the cells lose their ability to produce insulin. This condition is worsened in cases of obesity and lipotoxicity as the process of autophagy is hindered and the level of glucose in the blood rises without any check and control. One of the major causes of dysfunction of beta cells and related pathologies is the damage caused by the increased ER stress. In this way, obesity and its related stresses can target and destroy the beta cells of the pancreas and can trigger or aggravate diabetes and other metabolic pathologies.

The ablation of the autophagic process in adipose tissues tends to have beneficial effects against obesity. The process of adipogenesis is dependent on autophagy and the halt in the autophagic process due to obesity also decreases the adipogenic processes. This reduces the potential of an individual to gain a high amount of weight in obesity. So, loss of autophagy in adipose tissues is not so bad for obese individuals and acts as a protective mechanism against gaining extra weight.

Moreover, autophagy carries out the whitening of adipose tissue. The reduction in the number of mitochondria in the adipose tissue leads to the whitening of these tissues and is carried out via autophagic degradation of mitochondria. The decrease of autophagy allows the retention of mitochondria in white adipose tissues those results in an increase in the energy expenditure that consequently leads to the reduction of body weight.

The role of autophagy in each tissue is distinct, and the effect of obesity on the process of autophagy is also different. In some tissues, obesity and related stresses lead to the inactivation of the autophagic process, while in others, obesity leads to the induction of autophagy. The autophagic suppression in skeletal muscle, adipose tissues and liver, can have beneficial effects in obesity and related stresses.

ROLE OF AUTOPHAGY IN INCREASING LIFESPAN

The presence of biomarkers of aging including increased oxidative stress, damaged mitochondria and other organelles, and loss of membrane fluidity determine the quality of life and longevity. Lifestyle, diet, and exercise can detox our body of aging biomarkers and autophagy is the underlying mechanism of this cellular cleansing.

There are three primary ways to which the cytoprotective effects of autophagy is attributed; these include:

- The buffering of cellular stress according to the availability of nutrients by enhancing the provision of substrates for anabolic reactions and generation of energy to meet the needs of cellular metabolism,

- The removal of abnormal and harmful organelles, including uncoupled mitochondria, therefore removing oxidative stress from the cell, and

- The clearance of aggregates that are potentially toxic proteins.

These cytoprotective effects are regulated and enhanced by various cellular processes and immunogenic responses that help the body improve its functionality and achieve longevity. There are various autophagy-related genes that are related to longevity. The best-characterized pathway is the insulin/insulin-like growth factor 1 (IGF-1) pathway. This pathway includes other vital players of autophagy, including tyrosine kinase receptor, PtdIns 3-kinase and Akt/PKB.

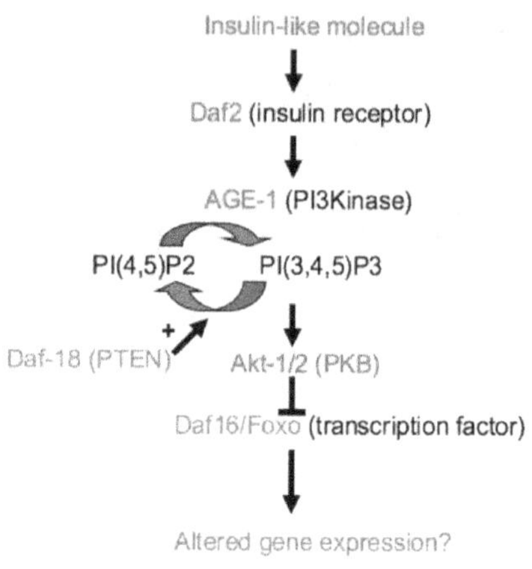

Figure 4. IGF-1 pathway

The longevity studies in nematode, *Caenorhabditis elegans*, suggests that the down-regulation of this cascade has positive effects on the longevity of worms - their lifespan was increased up to three hundred-fold. The inactivation of the IGF-1 pathway induces heat and oxidative stress resistance in these worm, which was found to be the contributing factor in increasing their lifespan. As we already know that Akt/PKB controls the functions of Tor, a suppressor of autophagy, the downregulation of Akt/PKB pathway in this experiment induces autophagy. It can be therefore concluded that autophagy has a significant role in the extension of lifespans.

As we age, there is a subsequent decrease in the process of autophagy which suggests that the two processes are correlated. Primarily, autophagy functions to protect the cell from oxidative damage by removing damaged mitochondria and facilitates other processes like replacement and repair of damaged DNA, lipids, and proteins. All these autophagy-related processes contribute to longevity and life-span expansion.

Mechanisms That Facilitate the Pro-Survival Attribute of Autophagy

Autophagy is a simple process that involves the degradation and removal of unwanted proteins and organelles from the body. The diverse cytoprotective effects of autophagy that lead to an increased life-span and healthy metabolism are attributed to the following processes:

- Proteostasis (Removal of abnormal proteins)

- Programmed cell death (Apoptosis)

- Inflammation

- Metabolism

- Hormesis

Proteostasis

The primary cytoprotective function of autophagy is its ability to remove toxic aggregates of protein that accumulate with aging. Various neurodegenerative disorders that are related to the process of aging, such as Parkinson's diseases and Alzheimer's disease (AD), are found to be caused by the accumulation of defective protein aggregates.

Unlike other processes that function to remove and eliminate defective proteins from the cell, autophagy can degrade large-sized protein aggregates.

Metabolism

Autophagy plays an essential role in various metabolic processes of the body. For instance, autophagy is involved in the lipid homeostasis of the body where it degrades lipid droplets present in cells. This process is known as lipophagy. Autophagy is involved in the process of gluconeogenesis that occurs in the liver where it regulates the level of glucose in the body. It also regulates the process of beta-oxidation of fatty acids and provides an alternative source of energy for the body when carbohydrates and glucose are absent or present in low amounts.

Programmed Cell Death

Activation of autophagy also mediates the process of programmed cell death, or apoptosis. Apoptosis is the regulator of cellular quality, and Beclin-1 mediates crosstalk with apoptotic machinery. This interaction ensures that there is no unnecessary removal of a cell when the damage within the cell can be cleared with autophagy. In this way, damaged mitochondria are removed from the cell, especially those comprising neuronal and muscle tissues, through the process of autophagy with no cellular loss by apoptosis. In this way, autophagy maintains the muscle mass of and neuron number in the body and provides protective effects on the skeletal muscle and nervous system.

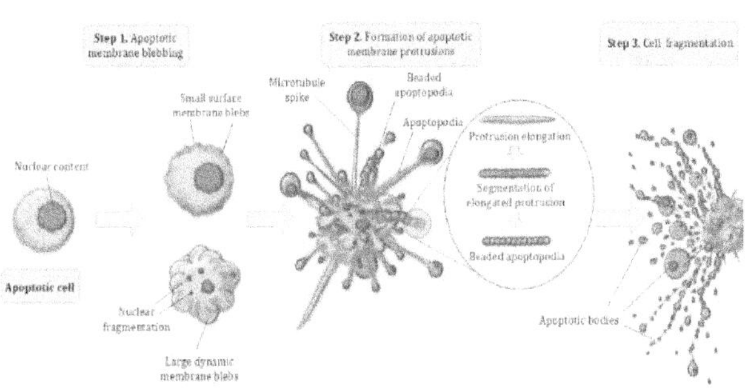

Figure 5. Apoptosis

Hormesis

A widely-studied phenomenon in toxicology is how the presence of a drug or a compound in lesser amounts is more beneficial and less toxic than in high amounts. Autophagy renders protective effects on the cell by carrying out detoxification and removes reactive oxygen species (ROS) that makes the cell more resistant to stresses that are related to age such as protein aggregates and oxidative damage.

Inflammation

The fact that cells become more inflamed with age has led to the development of a new term known as *inflammaging*. Autophagy plays a vital role in the elimination of inflammation from a cell. The production of pro-inflammatory cytokines in the leukocytes is reduced by the process of autophagy. Autophagy clears the cell from aging markers and ultimately reduces the inflammation from the body.

The Process of Aging and its Link with Autophagy

Aging is one of the strongest natural processes. It is characterized by a progressive decline in the repair and maintenance pathways that are integral to cellular homeostasis. The loss of cellular homeostasis leads to the accumulation of abnormal and dysfunctional organelles and biomolecules. These aberrant cellular components are misfolded, oxidized, aggregated and cross-linked, and have toxic effects on the cell structure and function. These defective molecules can interfere with the cell's functions directly or can compromise the functionality of other molecules and organelles, leading to detrimental effects on the cell. The homeostasis of cellular function is vital for the optimum functions of organs and organ systems. A progressive decrease in the efficacy of cellular homeostasis occurs as we age, leading to various diseases and eventually death.

Over the past century, however, our understanding of the biology of aging has increased. By way of advancements in the field of molecular biology, we have successfully explored the underlying molecular events of the aging process. Interestingly, it has been found that the rate of aging can be controlled by altering certain conserved cellular processes and signaling pathways in various organisms. These findings suggest that the process of aging can be utilized and manipulated as a therapeutic tool to combat various chronic and metabolic age-related disorders.

The processes and cellular pathways that have been found to modulate aging are conserved in various organisms, from yeasts to higher mammals, and have been collectively termed as conserved longevity paradigms. These paradigms will be discussed in the next section.

Melany Flores

Conserved Longevity Paradigms in Various Models

Recently, various genes have been identified that control the metabolic functions that influence the aging process in various model organisms. These models include the budding yeast, nematodes, fruit fly, and rodent models. The first studies were carried out in worms and showed that the positive effects of certain mutations in phosphoinositide 3-kinase (PI3K) and insulin/IGF-1–like receptors result in the extension of the organism's lifespan. There are more than 150 *C. elegans* genes that have been found to be involved in increasing their lifespan. And interestingly, most of these genes are part of metabolic signaling and endocrine processes.

The most important and widely studied longevity-associated pathways that primarily control metabolism and nutrient sensing are the insulin/IGF-1 and mTOR signaling cascades. The processes that affect the process of aging include dietary restriction, reproductive system signals and mitochondrial respiration. The list of processes and pathways which modulate aging and their effects on the process of autophagy are given in Table 7.

Table7. List of conserved longevity paradigms in relation with autophagy.

Sr #	Cellular Process	Changes	Effect on Autophagy	Effect on Longevity
1	Insulin/IGF-1 pathway	Decrease in insulin/IGF-1	Increase	Increase
2	mTOR signaling cascade	Decrease in signaling	Increase	Increase
3	Signals from reproductive system	Removal of germline	Increase	Increase
4	Mitochondrial respiration	Reduction in respiration rate	Increase	Increase
5	Dietary Restriction	Applying	Increase	Increase

The signaling cascades and processes that modulate the aging process, directly or indirectly, influence the process of autophagy. The involvement of these processes in regulation of autophagy and longevity make them a desirable candidate for research and provide insight into the complex process of aging. The longevity paradigms that are conserved in all eukaryotic organisms, from yeasts to humans are given below:

- Reduced TOR signaling

- Reduced insulin/IGF-1 signaling

- Germline removal

- Dietary Restriction

- Reduced mitochondrial respiration

Insulin/IGF-1 Signaling

Insulin/IGF-1 signaling is the primary pathway for the regulation of nutritional status in various animals. It plays an important role in the growth of organisms. The hormone insulin (or insulin-like growth factor; IGF-1) interacts with its receptor to activate a cascade of kinases and phosphatases. These include PI3K, and AKT that lead to the inhibition of the transcription factor FOXO. This transcription factor is involved in the stress-coping mechanism of the body and helps the organism to survive under unfavorable conditions.

The downregulation of insulin/IGF-1 in flies, worms, and mice has been found to be linked with an expansion of lifespan. Recent studies have shown that one genetic trait that was found to be common among long-lived humans, ie., centenarians, was the presence of gene mutations in the insulin/IGF-1 pathway. Hence, there exists an interesting relationship between the insulin/IGF-1 pathway and the process of aging – a relationship which is highly conserved.

TOR signaling

The TOR pathway regulates the process of aging. It is the member of the TOR PI3K-related kinase family. TOR is a nutrient-dependent pathway that is activated when a cell has enough nutrients and its metabolism is shifted towards cell division and growth. There are two forms of TOR complexes, TORC1 and TORC2. These complexes carry out distinct functions in the body by regulating various effector pathways. They mediate nutrient-based and mitogenic signals that carry out proliferation of the cell and determine the cell size. Inhibition of TORC1 has been found to be associated with aging delay. It is activated through the kinase AKT in the presence of amino acids.

The involvement of kinase AKT is a commonality between the insulin/IGF-1 and the TOR pathways. TORC1 leads to the activation of multiple anabolic processes. These include biogenesis of ribosome, initiation of translation, transport of nutrients, and inhibition of autophagy.

TOR signaling regulates the process of aging in many organisms. A reduction in the TOR activity can prolong the lifespan in yeast, flies, worms, and mice. There are two main processes that are influenced by TOR that effect longevity which are:

- Ribosomal protein S6 kinase (S6K) acts as a downstream target of TOR. The inhibition of S6K leads to the reduction of protein synthesis that leads to expansion of lifespan in worms, yeast, flies, and mice.

- TOR regulates the cellular recycling process of autophagy which mediates longevity.

Dietary restriction

Dietary restriction involves cutting down on nutrients while avoiding being malnourished. This approach is considered as the most robust methods that are currently being used to delay aging. This method has shown promising results in extending the lifespan of mice, hamsters, fish, yeast, invertebrates and apes. Advances in molecular biology have led to the findings that highlight the role of nutrient pathways, TOR signaling and insulin/IGF-1 in contributing to the longevity effects of dietary restriction.

Signals From the Reproductive System

Interestingly, there exists an inverse relationship exist between fertility and lifespan. Research shows that certain signals from the reproductive system have a positive effect on lifespan. By removing germ cells or germ line precursor cells from worms and flies, the lifespan of flies and worms were extended. However, the removal of the complete reproductive system or sterility did not have an effect of longevity which suggests that lifespan extension is not related to sterility but rather, the absence of signals which promote aging from germ line cells.

Reduced Mitochondrial Respiration

One of the most widely studied hallmarks of aging is the free-radical theory. The fact that the level of free radicals in the body is increased as we age can be one of the most obvious reasons for the cellular and organ dysfunction that is related to aging. Reactive oxygen species (ROS) can cause molecular damage to cells and cell components and can have deleterious effects on the body. One of the most important organelle of the cell, the mitochondria, plays an important role in the determination of ROS levels in the cell. ROS is produced during mitochondrial respiration and the reduction of mitochondrial respiration and reduced electron transport chain function can decrease the levels of ROS and increase lifespans in worms, yeast, flies, and mice. Studies in worms show that an increase in longevity is mediated by an upregulation of the mitochondrial unfolded protein response (UPR).

Aging is controlled in a highly conserved manner by various signaling pathways and processes. The primary objective in aging research is to find out whether these signaling pathways and processes that control lifespan have a common downstream mechanism. Current evidence suggests that autophagy, which is the cellular recycling process, is one of such mechanisms. Autophagy maintains cellular homeostasis and plays an important role in cleansing the cell from signs of aging and disease. In doing so, it helps in increasing the organism's lifespan.

ROLE OF AUTOPHAGY IN THE BODY

The process of autophagy occurs in a systematic manner in the body with varying rates in different parts and tissues of the body. As each organ of the body has different metabolic needs, the rate of autophagy also varies in each organ. The organs where the most efficient and elaborate system of autophagy occurs are the brain, liver, and muscles. Autophagy plays a different role in each of these organs and ensures the functioning, survival, and development of the cells of these tissues. The role of autophagy in these organs is distinct and will be discussed in the next section.

Autophagy and the Brain

As we know, autophagy is the primary housekeeping process of the cell. It can remove and recycle aged proteins, protein aggregates, and entire organelles. The most widely studied role of autophagy is in the brain cells where it provides remarkable neuroprotective effects.

Protein aggregates or inclusion bodies are common hallmarks of age-related neurodegenerative disorders. There is increasing evidence that these aggregates have toxic effects on the brain cells and interfere with neuronal function. These aggregates affect the hampering of axonal transport, integration of synapsis, regulation of transcription in neuronal cells, and mitochondrial function in the neurons, which lead to dysregulation of neuronal activity.

Neuroscientists have been focusing their research to find an effective treatment for neurodegenerative diseases to slow the age-related neural loss down and find way ways to clear the protein aggregates from neurons. Various studies imply that loss of autophagy increases the formation of inclusion body and triggers a neurodegenerative cascade. These findings highlight the role of autophagy as a built-in defense mechanism to cleanse the brain and nerve cells from inclusion bodies. It is becoming increasingly important to develop a better understanding of autophagy to better control the factors that influence healthy aging and neurodegeneration as well as to facilitate the development of new drugs and treatments.

Role of Autophagy in the Neurons

Various studies suggest that autophagy plays an important role in preventing the accumulation of inclusion bodies in the brain cells and renders a neuroprotective effect. The relationship between neuronal pathology and autophagy has been established by studying the effects of knockout mutations of the Atg5 and Atg7 genes in neuronal cells in mice. These genes are vital for the formation of autophagosomes and are therefore critical for the autophagic process. Deletion of these genes leads to increased cell death, progressive deficits in motor activity, and increases the formation of inclusion bodies. This shows that the loss of autophagy is enough to trigger a neurodegenerative cascade that compromises brain functions.

Mice with brain-specific Atg7 knock-out mutations showed an increased mortality rate, reduction in body size, loss of movement coordination and tremors, which are an indication of neurological faults. Lack of autophagy leads to neuronal loss; the most damaging type of neuronal loss is known as gliosis. Gliosis is characterized by the loss of pyramidal neurons, which is a diagnostic marker of neurodegenerative events.

The increase in age of Atg7- and Atg5-deficient mice led to an increase in ubiquitin-containing inclusion bodies in their neurons. The lack of autophagy was likely the reason for the formation and accumulation of inclusion bodies as normal autophagy functions to remove protein aggregates from the cell.

Neurodegenerative pathogenesis of brain-specific Atg5-deficient mice has been studied. These mice suffered from severe motor deficits, loss of Purkinje cells that regulate coordination and movement and accumulation of inclusion bodies. All these findings show that autophagy has a crucial role in the homeostasis and functioning of neurons. The optimal functioning of the autophagic system ensures the brain health, improves cognition, delay age-related memory loss and protects the brain from neurodegenerative diseases.

Autophagy and Successful Brain Aging

Thus far, we have established the importance of autophagy in preserving the health of the brain and nervous system. But there is also a definitive role of diet and calorie restriction in the protection of brain functions which can be attributed to the neuronal autophagic flux. Evidence from around 70 years of research on the link between calorie-restriction and autophagy provides fascinating insights on the role of CR-induced neuronal autophagy that protects the brain and increases the lifespan of humans. Therefore, following a low-calorie diet either by intermittent fasting or a fat-rich diet in combination with autophagy-inducing dietary supplements can significantly contributes to successful and healthy brain aging.

Autophagy and Liver

The self-eating process of autophagy plays an important role in the normal functioning of the liver. This catabolic pathway contributes to maintaining the homeostasis of the liver by regulating the energy needs of the cell as well as facilitating the removal of damaged organelles, misfolded proteins and droplets of lipids. In this way, autophagy has a major impact on hepatocytes. Other cells of the liver where autophagy plays an essential role include the hepatic stellate cells, endothelial cells and macrophages. Autophagy is a vital process for the health and proper functioning of the liver and any kind of error or abnormality in this process can lead to liver damage and dysfunction, which can also cause various diseases.

The most common type of liver diseases that occur due to the faulty autophagic system includes various storage diseases. As the liver is the metabolic hub of the body, it acts as a reservoir for different kind of metabolites. The inability to degrade and remove these metabolites from the liver cells due to malfunctioning of autophagy can cause the over-accumulation of these compounds in the cells of the liver and trigger various storage diseases. The most common types of liver diseases include Wilson's disease and alpha-1 antitrypsin deficiency. Several other kinds of liver disorders many also arise due to defects in autophagy; these include non-alcoholic steatohepatitis, hepatic carcinoma, chronic alcohol-related liver disease and acute injury of the liver tissues. The detrimental effects of autophagic errors make the process of autophagy a potential therapeutic strategy as by manipulating the process of autophagy and modulating its beneficial effects on the cell, we may be able to treat various liver diseases.

As discussed earlier, the liver is the primary metabolic and detoxifying organ in the body. As autophagy plays a significant role in the cleansing and cleaning process of cells, it ought to have a significant role in the liver. Apart from removing aggregates of abnormal proteins and damaged mitochondria, autophagy is also involved in the removal of swelling in hepatocytes.

A major inducer of liver autophagy is starvation. The major physiological functions of autophagy in the liver include β-oxidation of fatty acids, regulation of metabolic pathways such as gluconeogenesis and the formation of ketone bodies. Gluconeogenesis requires amino acids that are provided by degradation of proteins through the process of autophagy. The production of fatty acids is carried out mainly through the autophagic degradation of triglycerides that are stored in the form of lipid droplets. Autophagy regulates the level of very low-density lipoprotein (VLDL) particles in the serum through the process of lipophagy. This results in the release of fatty acids into the blood. Additionally, the autophagy process also plays an essential role in the maintenance of plasma glucose levels in neonates during starvation and fasting. Autophagy in the hepatocytes also provides protection against accumulation of fat in the liver.

Hepatoprotective Properties of Autophagy

Autophagy in the liver cells imparts an overall protective effect by providing protection against various kinds of stresses and diseases. Studies involving mice models with defective autophagy pathways are more vulnerable to liver injury from different toxic agents including alcohol, ischemia-reperfusion, and high levels of toxic free fatty acids. Macroautophagy protects against the death of liver cells by eliminating misfolded proteins, oxidized lipids, damaged mitochondria, and oxidative stress. It can provide the cells with the necessary nutrients to maintain cellular energy needs under conditions of injury and stress.

Autophagy and Hepatic Stellate Cells; Jekyll or Hyde for the Liver?

Hepatic stellate cells (HSC) are a type of mesenchymal cells that are present in the liver. They are located between the hepatocytes and blood vessels. HSCs are characterized by the presence of droplets of lipids and thin protrusions that extend around the blood vessels in the liver. HSCs play important roles in the physiology and fibrogenesis of the liver. Fibrogenesis of the liver is a cellular response to chronic liver injury. This can result from various metabolic disorders, alcohol consumption, or presence of chronic viral infections. Unlike the positive effects of autophagy on other liver cells, HSCs are prone to certain harmful effects of autophagy which can lead to liver damage and fibrosis. Autophagy is considered as a deleterious pathway in these fibrogenic cells.

It has been identified as the key player in the phenotypic switch of hepatic stellate cells from normal to fibrogenic phenotype as it causes a progressive loss of lipid droplets that contain retinoid. Catabolic action of autophagy degrades the lipids droplets via lipophagy. An increase in the catabolism of retinyl esters by autophagy leads to the generation of free fatty acids. These free fatty acids lead to the increased production of ATP, which acts as a trigger for the HSCs to acquire the fibrogenic profile. An increase in autophagic flux and the number of autophagic vacuoles in liver cells have been associated with an increase in LC3-II in human HSCs, proving the role of autophagy in inducing the fibrogenic activity of HSCs. Fibrosis of the liver tissue leads to chronic liver damage and loss of liver functions. It has been found that the primary triggers for the upregulation of autophagy in HSCs are ER and oxidative stress.

Various clinical interventions involving the inhibition of autophagy have resulted in the reduction of fibrogenic effects of HSCs. Inhibition of autophagy downregulates the fibrogenic properties of HSCs, which includes a reduction in cell proliferation rates and a reduced expression of fibrogenic genes. By using therapeutic measures, such as downregulation of the Atg5 or Atg7 genes, or by reducing oxidative stress, we can minimize the risks of liver fibrosis by the action of hepatic stellate cells. In this way, autophagy acts as a two-way sword for the liver cells, and it becomes a tricky question of whether it is the Jekyll or Hyde for the hepatocytes. Regardless, the importance of autophagy for the normal functioning and homeostasis of the liver is unquestionable.

Autophagy in the liver is an interesting process as apart from HSCs, it has positive effects on other types of liver cells including hepatocytes and macrophages. In fact, renders a hepatoprotective effect. While the death of a hepatocyte triggers the fibrogenic profile of HSCs, the process of autophagy prevents this trigger and protects the cell from fibrosis. Interestingly, in cases of α-1 antitrypsin deficiency, the induction of autophagy provides protection against hepatocyte death and fibrosis of the liver tissue. In epithelial cells, the process of autophagy proves to be a protective pathway against damage and fibrosis in various organs, including liver and kidneys. Thus, we can conclude that autophagy acts as a friend for macrophages and hepatocytes.

Melany Flores

Autophagy and Liver Regeneration

The liver is a special organ as it can regenerate itself and heal. Autophagy plays an important role in liver regeneration. It carries out the elimination of damaged proteins from the liver and maintains cellular energy needs; both these processes are crucial for tissue regeneration. The role of autophagy in elimination of damaged proteins and maintenance of intracellular energy highlights its importance in the process of liver regeneration.

Only a few studies have analyzed the role of autophagy in the regenerative process. It has been found that the removal of a small part of the liver led to an induction of autophagy in the early stages of the regeneration process.

Knockout mice with a specific deletion in the Atg5 or Atg7 genes in liver cells suffered from the accumulation of abnormal mitochondria and an impaired ability of liver regeneration when exposed to liver tissue removal. Hepatocytes with an abnormal autophagic system are unable to maintain the energy level that is required for cellular physiology and become aged. Macroautophagy provides protection against various defects in the regeneration process that may occur due to chronic liver injury.

Autophagy and Muscles

The skeletal muscles and neuronal tissues are the main sites of autophagy as the muscle cells contain the highest number of mitochondria and require an efficient system of organelle turnover. However, increased autophagy in muscle cells also makes them more prone to damage if any kind of abnormality arises in the process of autophagy.

Various muscular disorders have been linked with the abnormal accumulation of autophagic vacuoles. This group of muscular dysfunction is termed as autophagic vascular myopathies (AVMs). Two of the main disorders that affect humans due to errors in the autophagy system are Pompe disease and Danon disease. They are discussed below.

Danon Disease and Pompe Disease

The autophagic pathway plays a very important role in the homeostasis of the skeletal muscles. It provides a cellular quality-check system that ensures the degradation of proteins and removal of old organelles. The autophagosomes function to engulf damaged organelles, cytoplasm and protein aggregates. This autophagosome then attaches to lysosomes for the degradation of its cargo. Lysosomes are an important part of the autophagic process and any kind of dysfunction in the lysosomal role in autophagy can have serious health effects.

The importance of lysosomes in the muscle is highlighted by the important role it plays in a group of muscular diseases. These disorders are caused by the accumulation of autophagic vacuoles in the cell due to impaired lysosomal function. The accumulation of autophagosomes proves to be toxic to the cell and hinders the normal cell physiology and function. This group of disorders is referred to as autophagic vacuolar myopathies (AVMs). These include Danon disease (DD), Pompe/glycogen storage disease type II (GSDII) and X-linked myopathy with excessive autophagy (XMEA).

Danon disease is an X-linked dominant disease. It is characterized by an anomaly of lysosome-associated membrane protein 2 (LAMP2). Patients with DD suffer from cardiomyopathy, weakness of muscles and mental retardation.LAMP2 carries out the maturation of autophagosomes and aids in the process of endosomal fusion. A lack of this gene causes failure of autophagosomal fusion to the lysosome, which results in accumulation of these autophagic vesicles in the muscle cells. This leads to muscular weakness and deterioration of mental health.

Pompe disease is characterized by deficiency of lysosomal enzyme known as acid alpha-glucosidase. The deficiency of this enzymecauses abnormality in the degradation and removal of glycogen. The accumulation of glycogen occurs in various tissues, however, the most harmful effects have been observed in the skeletal and cardiac muscles.

Autophagy and the Vascular System

Like in other cells and tissues, autophagy plays a protective role in vascular endothelial cells that are prevalent in our veins and arteries. In the vascular endothelial cells, autophagy carries out a crucial role by providing protection against various pathophysiological stimuli. These include exposure to reactive oxygen species, hypoxia, end products of glycation, oxidized low-density lipoprotein, and lipopolysaccharides. Various natural compounds that have antioxidant and anti-inflammatory activity, such as vitamin D, curcumin, and resveratrol, can promote autophagy in ECs. The use of these compounds helps to protect against oxidative stress and endothelial inflammation and injury.

Autophagy in Atherosclerosis

Atherosclerosis is a chronic disease of the arteries. It is characterized by inflammation of the arterial wall and has high mortality rates all over the world, and especially in developing countries. Atherosclerosis occurs due to the production and accumulation of lipid-containing plaques in the vessel wall. It is one of the most prevalent age-related diseases. Other risk factors that lead to an increased risk of developing atherosclerosis include hypertension, smoking, obesity, diabetes and hypercholesterolemia.

Recent evidence suggests that the presence of a dysfunctional autophagic system is the primary cause of atherosclerosis. The vascular cells fail to trigger autophagy when they are exposed to oxidative stress, cytokines and oxidized lipids that are present in plaque. This tends to have a damaging effect on vascular health as the presence of plaque leads to hardening of arteries and a loss of elasticity. As autophagy is a catabolic process, the formation of atherosclerotic plaque should be solved by this process. However, defects in autophagy lead to the failure of removal of plaques from the arteries and it has therefore been postulated that autophagy plays a main role in modulation of atherogenesis and in the stability of atherosclerotic plaque. It has been found that defective autophagy promotes the process of cell death and apoptosis in macrophages. It promotes premature senescence in vascular smooth muscle cells (VSMCs) and both apoptosis and senescence in epithelial cells. By developing a better understating of the defects of the autophagic process in these three types of cells, we can model the autophagic process for therapeutic purposes and find new autophagy-based cures for vascular diseases.

METHODS TO MONITOR AUTOPHAGY

Several methods have been developed to monitor and measure the rate and flux of autophagy in cells. These methods have become widely used and have gained great importance owing to the significance of autophagy in the field of research and therapeutic sciences. Recent advancements in microscopic and molecular biology have led to the development of various methods that have high accuracy. Some of the widely used methods for the measurement and monitoring of autophagy are discussed below:

1) Staining Methods and Microscopy

- Monod-ansylcadaverine (MDC)

- LysoTracker

- Acridine orange

2)Screening of autophagic markers and immunohistochemistry

- LC3

3) Autophagic flux

- Sequestration assay

- Use of radio labeled assay

- Ape1 (aminopeptidase 1) maturation assay

1). Staining Methods and Microscopy

The acidotropic stains, including MDC (Monodansylcadaverine), LysoTracker and acridine orangeare commonly used for the labeling of acidic compartments in cells. These include autolysosomes, endosomes, and lysosomes. An increase in these organelles can be easily monitored by using these stains and subsequent visualization through electron microscopy. As membranes are easily stained by these acidotropic stains, the double-membrane of autophagosomes are proven to be the most prominent structures for monitoring the rate and level of autophagy in any cell.

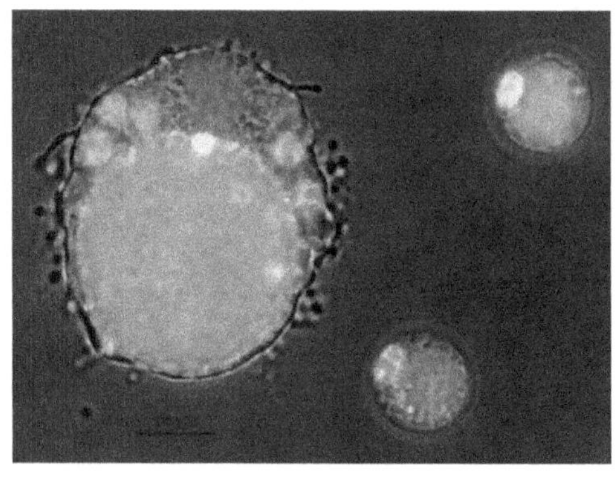

Figure 6. Lysotracker stain

2)Screening of Autophagic Markers and Immunohistochemistry

Another method for the detection of the level of autophagy in a cell includes screening for the presence of certain autophagy-related proteins or autophagic markers. One of the most widely used proteins is a homolog of Atg8 in yeast, termed as LC3. LC3 is a microtubule-associated protein and is one of the most efficient autophagy markers. The level of LC3 in a cell is equivalent to its level of autophagic processes. There are two predominant forms of LC3 protein in the cell, LC3-II and LC3-I. The level of LC3-I is typically high in normal cells, while LC3-II levels are only increased in a cell during autophagy. The relative changes of LC3-II and I provide a clear indication of the autophagy levels in a cell.

There are two ways through which the level of LC3-I and LC3-II levels and their interchangeability is analyzed to monitor the level of autophagy. These include western blotting and immunofluorescence or immunohistochemistry. During western blotting, the level of LC3-II in the cell can be visualized on a gel using cell extracts and a suitable marker for the protein. For immunological analysis, antibodies against LC3-II can be used for detecting the level of autophagy marker in a cell. Another method is the fluorescence methods, where fusion of a fluorescent marker to the N-terminus of LC3 can be used to monitor the sub-cellular localization of this protein and thereby, the induction of autophagy in a cell.

These methods are used to determine the steady-state measurements of autophagy in the cell. To determine the efficiency of the autophagy process in certain cells and at specific conditions, it is necessary to use other methods which can measure the autophagic flux. Autophagic flux is determined by analyzing the rate of lysosomal delivery of the cargo and its degradation in the lysosome. This is a vital feature of the autophagy process and its analysis aids us in determining the factors which affect the process of autophagy.

3)Autophagic flux

There are different methods that can be used to monitor autophagic flux. Sequestration assay is one of the most widely used methods for this purpose. In this method, an artificial cargo, [3H]-raffinose, is injected into the cytoplasm of the cell. This cargo is sequestered and transferred into an insoluble fraction through the formation of autophagosome. The rate at which [3H]-raffinose is transferred to autophagic vesicles and removed from the cytoplasm is monitored and autophagic flux is determined.

Another method to monitor the autophagic flux is by analyzing the rate of protein degradation. This method involves the use of radiolabeled proteins. The degradation of proteins into amino acids will result in the release of radioactive amino acids into the cytoplasm. The level of radioactivity will be proportional to the rate of protein degradation by autophagy.

The Ape1 (aminopeptidase 1) maturation assay is also used to determine the autophagic flux in the yeast cell. It involves the autophagic conversion of Ape1 into its mature form in the autophagic vacuoles that are equivalent to the lysosome in mammalian cells.

Other strategies to measure autophagic flux include the monitoring of turnover of LC3-II, or the removal of autophagic substrates from the cell.

WHEN DO THE RESULTS OF AUTOPHAGY START TO SHOW?

Autophagy is a highly regulated and complex process. To get the full benefits of this process, it is important that we adopt a certain routine and then follow it strictly. By following a strict autophagic routine, one can start seeing the results of autophagy in around two weeks.

In one study, based on finding the positive effects of autophagy, they determined the level of health biomarkers, such as skin complexion, body/mass index (BMI) etc., in the body. It was found that by eating certain autophagy inducing foods and following an exercise routine for eight weeks, the individuals felt more active, energetic and healthy.

As autophagy is induced in response to stressful conditions, one must trick his body into believing there is stress. The study used the following key autophagy-activators that function perfectly to induce stress in the body:

- Low-carb and high-fat diet

- Excluding proteins completely from the diet

- Fasting for two days a week or trying other types of intermittent fasting

- Doing high-intensity interval training exercises

AUTOPHAGY—THE BEST BODY DETOX REGIMEN

If you need a detox, you don't always have to go with liquid kale and other stuff that doesn't taste good. Autophagy is a natural way through which our body cleanses itself. It helps in maintaining the quality of cells and its organelles, reduces inflammation, and keeps your body running in tip-top shape. Autophagy is essentially a fine-tuning mechanism or the housekeeping staff of our body.

Autophagy and intermittent fasting together provide the perfect detox regimen. They help to clear our body of harmful toxins, burn extra weight, and renew our body right at the molecular level. The detoxification effects of autophagy and intermittent fasting are amazing. Together they promote the anti-aging process and lead to longevity.

PRECAUTIONS RELATED TO AUTOPHGY

Autophagy is an amazing process that has many beneficial effects on the body. However, to enjoy the benefits of autophagy to the fullest, it is necessary to follow the authentic and safe methods of inducing autophagy.

While practicing fasting to induce autophagy, it is advisable to fast with good and healthy intervals, rather than long-term fasting.

If you are suffering from certain health problems and are using medications for it, it is advisable to consult with a doctor before adopting any autophagy-related routine, such as fasting, high-intensity exercising or dietary restrictions. People suffering from hypoglycemia, hypertension or diabetes, or those with a family history of these diseases, must take precautions before going for autophagy inducing routines. Women who are pregnant or are breastfeeding infants must not try intermittent fasting. If you are a beginner to fasting, it is advisable to start with a relatively easy approach called crescendo fasting which involves a 12-hour fast routine.

If you are opting for calorie restriction as an inducer of autophagy, then it is advisable that you keep a complete check on your diet and make sure all the essential macro and micronutrients are included in the diet. This will ensure a balanced diet and will protect you from malnutrition.

While doing high intensity exercises, we should take care and listen to our body. One should not push himself beyond his limits and should allow his muscles and body to heal and repair before exercising again. It is also advisable to follow recommendations from a professional trainer.

So, the takeaway message is that it is necessary to stay safe while aiming to achieve certain goals with autophagy. Autophagy has a lot to offer for the betterment and well being of our health, but there are certain notions and protocols that we should follow to avoid any kind of undesired outcomes.

FUTURE PERSPECTIVES REGARDING AUTOPHAGY AND ITS THERAPEUTIC ROLE

The Unanswered Questions

The relationship between food and autophagy has increased the importance of nutrition and dietary choices. Furthermore, the role of dietary modifications in disease prevention has become increasingly important. Various health-promoting dietary components and their mechanism of action on the physiology of the body have been identified and their effects on autophagy have been widely studied. Autophagy is upregulated by consuming certain foods and has been used as a key therapeutic tool for the treatment of neurodegenerative diseases and cancer. However, the exact role of dietary components in the regulation of autophagy and autophagic flux and the diverse effects of autophagy in the body needs to be further investigated. Moreover, the exact role of autophagy in cancer needs more extensive research as multiple studies suggest that under certain circumstances, autophagy acts as a suppressor of tumorous cells, while in others it aggravates the tumor. It is necessary to determine when autophagy is beneficial and when it is non-beneficial, so that we can effectively manipulate the autophagic process and develop autophagy-inducing drugs for improving human health. There are some unanswered questions regarding the autophagic process in relation to dietary components that may govern its effectiveness in therapeutic field. For instance:

1. Where, when and how are the autophagy-inducing food components metabolized in the cell?

2. Will the nutrients survive in the human body in an active form for long enough to affect the autophagic process?

3. Will the metabolites of these nutrients also be biologically active or have the potential to influence autophagy?

4. What should be the effective and safe concentration of these nutrients that one needs to consume to trigger autophagy?

5. Will the effect of these food components be systematic or targeted? Will the nutrients only interact and affect the cells of the gastrointestinal tract, or will they be able to enter the blood and reach other parts of the body?

6. Is it necessary to prepare, store, and consume the food in a specific manner to obtain their autophagic benefits?

7. What kind of interactions will these compounds have with pharmaceutical drugs?

It is important to identify every compound that is present in the foods we eat and understand their effects on the body. It is also important to understand how all the components present in our diet could affect autophagy and other cellular processes. If we use dietary components and food supplements that induce autophagy for therapeutic purposes, it is necessary that we understand the interaction of food components with each other as well as their overall effects on the body. For example, if we use the autophagy-inducing diet for treating breast cancer, we should be able to make a solid hypothesis about the effects of such a diet on the hormone levels in the body. Such diverse implications of diet, governed by physiology as well as genetics, makes autophagy-induced therapy a tricky matter. We should utilize methods such as personalized-therapy and nutritional-healing so that we can get the most out of the autophagic process for therapeutic purposes.

CONCLUSION AND FINAL THOUGHTS

Autophagy was initially identified as a responder of cellular stress, but with increasing research and studies it has been established that it is a much more complex and beneficial process of the mammalian physiology. Autophagy plays an important role in the maintenance of normal physiological roles and contributes to regulating the development, growth, and aging of mammals. It is the natural cleansing process of the cell and rids the body of signs of aging and disease.

Autophagy plays a significant role in a variety of disorders and diseases. It is a complex process, and its exact role in various diseases remains controversial. As we age, the process of autophagy gradually diminishes, which is manifested by a decrease in the formation of autophagosomes or the inappropriate fusion of these vacuoles with the lysosomes. In the case of neurodegenerative disorders, the accumulation of certain proteins is attributed to the failure in the autophagic elimination of these toxic proteins. Various lysosomal disorders are attributed to the dysfunction of the autophagic process that leads to the accumulation of lipid droplets in the lysosomes. Autophagy plays a very confusing role in cancer, where it acts as tumor suppressor in the initial stages but as a tumor promoter by protecting the cancer cells from the immune system. Moreover, autophagy positively and negatively regulates various kinds of muscular and heart disorders respectively. On the other hand, the induction of the autophagic pathway plays an important role in fighting and removing foreign pathogens. It is a vital part of innate immunity. The effect of downregulation of autophagy in obesity and related stresses varies and is highly tissue-dependent.

Autophagy operates locally and systematically in various tissues of the body. It is involved in the development and growth of tissues in different ways. When autophagy is impaired, the differentiating tissues undergo deleterious effects and the whole physiology of the body is disturbed. Autophagic errors lead to various metabolic and chronic disorders as well as cancers, which can be life-threatening.

Various regimens have been adopted to artificially induce autophagy in the body. These approaches help in the upregulation of autophagy to gain benefits like anti-aging, detox, weight loss, and longevity. It also provides protection against neurodegenerative diseases, chronic illnesses, diabetes, hypertension and cardiovascular diseases.

Further research is required to understand the systemic role of autophagy in the mammalian life cycle. This will provide us with a better understanding of developmental biology in relation to the process of autophagy, which will aid us in finding new targets for the treatment of complex and chronic diseases. We need to utilize the basic scientific knowledge that we have about autophagy for therapeutic purposes. Because of the extremely diverse role of autophagy in biochemical and signaling pathways, its importance is greatly increased from a clinical perspective. The role of autophagy in the manifestation of metabolic disorders, neurodegenerative diseases, aging, inflammatory diseases and cancer have made it an ideal candidate to be explored for its therapeutic and diagnostic implications in managing various diseases.

I hope this book provided you with all the useful information that you wanted to have. Don't forget to write a short review of the book on Amazon if you liked it!

✱✱✱